DR. ZIZMOR'S
SKIN CARE
BOOK

DR. ZIZMOR'S SKIN CARE BOOK

by Jonathan Zizmor, M. D.

with John Foreman

Holt, Rinehart and Winston · New York

Copyright © 1977 by Jonathan Zizmor and John Foreman
All rights reserved, including the right to reproduce
this book or portions thereof in any form.

Published simultaneously in Canada by
Holt, Rinehart and Winston of Canada, Limited.

Grateful acknowledgment is made to *Cutis* for permission to
reproduce the chart that appears on pp. 178–180.

Portions of this book have previously appeared in
Family Health and *Mademoiselle* magazines.

Library of Congress Cataloging in Publication Data

Zizmor, Jonathan.
 Dr. Zizmor's skin care book.

 Includes index.
 1. Skin—Care and hygiene. I. Foreman, John,
1945–   joint author. II. Title. [DNLM: 1.
Dermatology—Popular works. WR100 Z82d]
RL87.Z58   616.5′05   76–29920
ISBN Hardbound: 0–03–017846–0
ISBN Paperback: 0–03–021471–8

First Edition
Designer: Mary M. Ahern
Printed in the United States of America
2 4 6 8 10 9 7 5 3 1

Contents

v

Introduction

You are about to learn the mysteries of dermatology. Don't worry, it won't be confusing. A great deal of effort has been devoted to making this book understandable and easy to use—while in the privacy of your own home. The book contains over one hundred step-by-step regimens to help you achieve more beautiful skin, no matter what your skin type. It will guide you through cosmetic shopping, teach you how to care for your hair and nails, and show you how to analyze your skin and tailor your daily routines to enhance your appearance. It will even explain when to get professional help, and how and where to find it.

Every beauty regimen in this book rests on a granite foundation of medical fact. What's more, the medical reasons behind every piece of advice are all clearly explained. Each chapter is like a visit to the dermatologist and an afternoon at a chic skin care salon rolled into one. What you'll learn in these pages is a result of many years of teaching dermatology and maintaining a private practice in New York City. Now I'm sharing my knowledge with you in a format that's easy and (I hope) entertaining as well.

The first part of this skin care book presents an overview of health and beauty. It's a compilation of many years of medical practice. Here are the answers to the most frequently asked questions in dermatology—questions about makeup, cosmetic surgery, bathing, beauty masks, diet, perspiration, sun exposure, and so forth.

Next comes "The Do-It-Yourself Skin Test," one of the most unique features of this book. You've probably seen tests like this in magazines, or possibly you've been to one of the better skin salons and taken one. Now you'll discover not only the reasons behind all the questions but also what the answers really mean. At the end of this test, you will have profiled your own skin type and compiled a reference list of page numbers that will enable you to look up specific advice for your own skin type.

Step-by-step improvement regimens make up the rest of the text. Whether you're overly oily, overly dry, losing your hair, wrinkling with age, have large pores, cracked lips, acne, and so on, there is help and advice for you.

Finally, in the Formulary you'll find alphabetical lists, divided by function, of all the many medications and preparations recommended in the book. In addition, numerous products that don't appear in the text but are just as good as those mentioned are listed in the Formulary. This is not meant to be an exhaustive catalogue of every medical preparation on the market. Its function is to give you a useful list that contains adequate alternatives.

Although this book is primarily for women, there is

help for everyone in these pages. Female or male, young or old, dry or oily, black or white, if you have a normal skin problem, you'll find ways to help yourself.

Before we start, I want to explain two terms that appear frequently throughout the text. The first is the abbreviation OTC, which stands for "over the counter." The difference between an OTC drug and a prescription drug is that the latter requires a prescription written by a medical doctor. In contrast, an OTC medication can be purchased by anyone and no prescription is necessary. The other term is "topical." Medicine that's applied "topically" is rubbed onto the surface of the skin, as opposed to "systemic" medications that enter the system usually as pills and do their work from the inside.

I think you're ready to begin now. And when you're finished with the book, I hope you'll look like a million dollars!

DR. ZIZMOR'S
SKIN CARE
BOOK

1

Great Skin Secrets of Yesterday and Today

I thought it would be interesting to start with a few beauty secrets from the past, particularly since the ancients had some pretty innovative ideas about personal appearance, although admittedly, they were mostly interested in good makeup. Today we live longer and we're naturally more worried about wrinkles and aging. And whereas our forebears lived in more natural surroundings and ate more natural foods, we live in overheated houses, sit in the sun too much, and consume quantities of chemicals (added to prepared and dietetic foods) undreamed of in earlier ages.

This is not to say that the practices and remedies of ancient or vanished cultures aren't applicable today. You'd be surprised how many things have cropped up as "new" discoveries after languishing unnoticed for thousands of years. Here's a good example: Babylonian women kept the skin of their legs soft and supple by wrapping their legs in urine-soaked towels, a practice longed ascribed purely to Babylonian madness—at least until the discovery of urea, a close chemical relative of uric acid. Urea is a hydrophilic, which means it attracts and holds moisture. Today it's used in excellent nonoily moisturizing products (notably Aquacare and Carmol) that moisturize the skin without clogging pores or causing pimples.

The ancients, if I may for convenience lump them together under that title, have taught modern doctors and cosmetologists many other things. Saltwater baths, for instance, are used to combat eczema today, just as they have for ages. A medication called psoralin is currently used in combination with sunlight to treat psoriasis, but it was also used for the same purpose in the Egypt of the pharaohs. And as for all the new lemon-freshened shampoos on the market, ancient people in the Mediterranean were degreasing their hair with lemons and oranges thousands of years ago. Citric juice, incidentally, is the ultimate "nonalkaline" substance, since it is all the way at the acid end of the pH scale.

Today's resurgence of interest in herbs and natural foods is almost like a throwback to biblical times, when people were "anointed" with scents and oils and ate nothing artificial. As far as beauty and skin were concerned, the emphasis back then was on temporary measures to make you look and feel good for a limited time. Women went in for masks and mud baths and didn't kid themselves that these measures would prevent aging or correct existing skin damage. After her facial, the beauty of several thousand years ago would paint herself with berry stains and be ready for an evening of intrigue. Everything she used was organic, but there was no expectation that it would make over her skin.

Certainly one of our great beauty legacies is the recognition of two chemical categories: humectants and rubifactants. Substances from these two categories have been used throughout the ages and are still used today to help skin problems that stem from excessive dryness or oiliness.

A humectant seals moisture into the skin. It's usually sticky and occlusive (pore clogging), and is applied as a mask to a face that's been patted with clean water. Elizabeth Arden does it essentially the same way Cleopatra did. The mask is allowed to dry and seal moisture in. When it's peeled off, a few superficial layers of cells come off, along with the tops of blackheads. The face feels refreshed and invigorated, even wrinkles look temporarily better. But the hands of time have not been turned back.

Rubifactants are plants and herbs that irritate the skin and cause it to peel. This mild peeling is very helpful for people with oily skin whose pores are constantly becoming clogged. Pores clogged with excessive oil constitute the primary cause of acne. The slight irritation and mild peeling that stems from application of a rubifactant will strip off excess oil, blackhead tops, and oil plugs and give the face a healthy, clean, and ruddy glow.

The acne soaps of today, such as Fostex, are in effect modern rubifactants.

Armed with a little knowledge, you can give yourself a humectant or rubifactant facial for something like half a dollar. If you have dry skin and hanker for a good humectant mask, here are a few ideas: The basis of your mask could be egg whites, honey, cactus (any kind), or cucumbers, to name only a few. Take your chosen substance (minus spines or skin) and put it in a blender together with a half-cup of skim milk, a thickener (plain Knox gelatin works well), and two cubes of ice. (Use the "puree" setting on the blender.) When your concoction has thickened, darken the room, put on soft music, and paint the face from chin to forehead with a sable makeup brush, leaving plenty of room around the eyes, mouth, and nostrils. For extra zest, you can add a drop of something like oil of wintergreen (my personal favorite) to the blender, being certain not to choose an oil to which you're allergic.

When the face is painted, relax and let the mask harden for half an hour, then peel it off. It should come off pretty much in one piece. After a quick warm-water wash you will feel terrific, have freshly moisturized skin, and look quite wonderful for the evening. I want also to recommend the Chinese herbal mask, described in Dr. Robert Alan Franklin's excellent book *The Art of Staying Young*. Again it's made with a blender, this time filled with bay and eucalyptus leaves, plus four ounces of liquid tea that need not be Chinese. Puree and paint it on as above.

If you have oily skin problems, you might want to

try a natural rubifactant treatment. Pineapple, papaya, yogurt, and herbs such as juniper, mint, pine, and rosemary are all good choices. Crush or chop any of these and rub on small amounts with the fingers until you feel slight irritation. (If you're using one of the herbs, buy it in essential oil form.) Wait about five minutes, then wash the face with a superfatted soap like Lowila Cake or Basis Soap. The result is akin to a very mild face peel that removes oil and blackhead tops and makes wrinkles look temporarily better.

You can also make a rubifactant mask by using the humectant recipe given above, substituting a rubifactant for the humectant. But be very careful not to over-irritate the face, lest you look sunburned instead of attractively ruddy.

While we are on the subject of oily faces, you might try washing with freshly squeezed lemon or orange juice from time to time instead of soap. This is an excellent way to degrease the skin without affecting the acid mantle many doctors claim is important to healthy skin.

I'll end this chapter with another old trick that nicely complements your freshened and beautified complexion. Nothing can make hair grow more quickly, no matter what anybody says, but you can make your hair look a lot thicker and richer by adding protein to the outside surfaces of the hair. To do it simply, add either egg whites or powdered plain gelatin, along with a small amount of lemon juice, to your shampoo. The lather will feel thicker, and your hair will have a lot more body.

2

The Diet for Your Skin

The key to good skin is a balanced diet. But don't think you're eating a balanced diet if you merely supplement it daily with fistfuls of vitamins. I know this seems to fly in the face of the current emphasis in nutrition therapy. The vogue these days is megavitamin therapy, massive dosages in quantities that sometimes exceed a year's normal intake in a matter of days.

Adequate vitamins absorbed through proper diet are a prerequisite of good skin. I commonly see patients with bad acne conditions who turn out to be consuming unnatural amounts of vitamins or health foods such as wheat germ. The first problem stems from the fact that many multivitamins and mineral supplement pills contain heavy dosages of iodides and bromides. These substances are known to cause pustular eruptions in the skin. Sad to say, very many health foods, such as kelp and wheat germ, are just as bad. Kelp is loaded with iodides, and wheat germ is extremely androgenic. Androgenic substances stimulate the sebaceous oil glands to secrete excessive amounts of oil, a condition that can bring on an acne flare-up. (See Chapter 7 for a full discussion of the causes of acne.)

Few people seem to realize that vitamins are not *all* good. It's also seldom remembered that the body naturally speeds up the elimination of anything that enters it in unnaturally large amounts. Thus, taking excessive amounts of a particular vitamin can possibly lead to an actual deficiency. In the case of Vitamin C, if that doesn't happen, another adverse effect might be bladder stones, whose appearance has been linked to too much Vitamin C.

Medical literature abounds with other examples of the negative side effects of vitamin therapy. Topically applied Vitamin E oil, very much a fad these days, can cause allergic reactions or acne. There's no proof that it speeds healing. Too much Vitamin A can yellow the skin (especially the palms) and lead to uncomfortable dryness. Pity the poor Eskimo who's had to dine on polar bear liver, a substance so rich in Vitamin A that it's been known to be fatal!

The point is not that vitamins are bad but that it is not uncommon to take an overdose. Vitamins are easy to get and just as easily abused. Certainly if you're young and battling natural acne, you're foolish to take them. And if you're older and seeking the key to longevity, don't forget that two leading health-food writers have died untimely deaths recently, at ages far less than my smoking, drinking, swearing, ninety-year-old Aunt Sally.

Keep vitamins in perspective; life span is much more a matter of genes.

While healthy skin requires a diet that provides all vitamins in moderation, what's much more important is calories. With insufficient calories, the skin will literally break down. Dieting for weight loss is a good idea, and more of us should do it. But crash dieting is a terrible idea. Impossibly rapid weight loss usually turns out to be temporary, and not particularly good for overall health. What's worse, there are definite hazards connected with the use of diet pills that directly affect the skin. Water pills, for example, cause dehydration that makes skin flaky and wrinkled. They may make you itch like crazy—especially if the environment is dry. Thyroid pills are no better. They speed up the metabolism so that calories are more rapidly consumed, but at the same time they make the skin soft and boggy, flushed and filled with fluid. These pills also encourage a velvety hair growth on the arms. Amphetamines can speed a person up to the point where hormone levels become unbalanced; hair can fall out, you might miss your menstrual period and might even get a bad case of acne. And as for human gonadotrophic injections, well, with luck you've never even heard of them. The FDA warns against them in any event, so you probably won't be able to subject yourself to these large hormone shots that knock your own hormonal levels out of whack and generally bring on large acne breakouts and hair loss.

My advice for dieters is to be sensible. Eat less, count calories, and don't rush. I also know that this simple advice is not easy to follow. Naturally slim people in good physical condition look that way because they don't overeat and they do get exercise. Life for most of us includes too much liquor, hardly any exercise, crazy eating schedules, and quantities of cardboard food. These pumped-up products are often bereft of food value but are flavored and marketed so ingeniously as to make us yearn to gobble "the whole thing." If you're going to reverse the process of self-bloating, expect inconveniences. Successful dieting means cutting out friendly drinks or counting their calories in your day's allotment. Primarily, you have to bring order and more than a little dullness into your diet. Don't skip meals, always choose broiled rather than fried foods, eat raw vegetables, and do without butter sauce. Remember that even those trendy eat-all-you-want diets inevitably follow up the rapid weight loss phase with a maintenance period that boils down to nothing more than calorie counting. You might just as well be sensible and start counting right from the beginning.

I'm going to spare you the boring recital of what all the vitamins supposedly do for you. And you already know that a balanced diet will provide adequate vitamin levels. But I do want to talk for just a moment about Vitamin F, the name lately given to "essential fatty acids." These fatty acids control skin metabolism and the rate of surface-cell shedding. Skin, incidentally, grows from the inside out, and as new layers form below, old layers continually shed off the top. Vitamin F is essential to regular healthy maintenance of this basic body system. Major sources are whole milk, cereal grains, and vegetable oils (corn, safflower, and olive).

Diets that eliminate these substances are, by definition, bad for the skin.,

You can get Vitamin F from lard or the white fat on meat too, but these are saturated fats. I'm sure you are aware of the desirability of unsaturated fats, which is loudly and constantly proclaimed via television commercials. While essential fatty acids are found in both saturated and unsaturated fats, a diet heavy in saturated fats will lead to trouble. Saturated fats will gradually clog blood vessels, usually lead to obesity, and sometimes cause heart attacks. The fatty acids in unsaturated (or polyunsaturated) foods don't seem to do the same thing. In fact, unsaturated fatty acids appear to exchange places with saturated fatty acids already in your system. So you can maintain good skin metabolism and reduce your body's level of potentially dangerous saturated fats at the same time.

The Diet That's Kind to Your Skin

Here is a do-it-yourself diet that is just as good for weight gain as for weight loss. First, to determine how many calories you need to maintain your current weight, multiply your weight by 15. To go up or down, adjust daily intake by adding or subtracting 10 percent. Whatever you do, don't hurry. And don't cheat either. Get yourself a little calorie-counting book at a drugstore and keep track. *The Brand Name Calorie Counter*, edited by Corinne Netzer and published by Dell, and *The Dictionary of Calories and Carbohydrates*, edited by

Barbara Kraus and published by New American Library, are my favorites. The more experienced you become, the less you'll need the book. To start you off on good eating habits, I suggest you try the diet given below, although there are scores of substitutions you can make.

A last word of advice in the skin department: beware in general of blushing foods—hot, peppery things, also caffein and alcohol—as they cause vasodilation (a natural enlargement of the blood vessels to ventilate out excess body heat). Diets consistently heavy in blushing foods cause permanently enlarged capillaries that are not attractive on the skin's surface.

Breakfast

Small glass of juice or a piece of citrus fruit (be careful; orange juice has lots of calories)

1 or 2 soft-boiled eggs or 1 egg fried or scrambled

A piece of toast with polyunsaturated margarine and jelly (jelly used in moderation is not very caloric)

Tea or coffee (black or with milk)

Note: Avoid bacon (too caloric, too fatty; contains nitrates which some doctors link to cancer); at most make it a once-a-week treat.

Rush Alternative: French cruller (sweet, not too heavy, and only 150 calories!); tea or coffee (black or with milk). But avoid instant chemical cubes and powders (too caloric, too many vitamins, too expensive!).

Mid-Morning Snack (for those who must): A citrus fruit (e.g., an orange or half a grapefruit); a teaspoon of corn oil—for Vitamin F—or save the corn oil for your salad.

Lunch

Tuna-, egg-, or chicken-salad sandwich (hold the mayo) with a pickle

Cole slaw (never potato salad)

Slice of fruit pie (if you can afford the calories, but not à la mode in any event)

Tea or coffee (black or with milk; try not to drink any coffee after 1 P.M. lest the caffein make you too jittery)

Quality Alternatives: If circumstances prohibit a sandwich lunch, then have broiled chicken or fish, a leafy salad, and don't eat bread. Avoid hamburgers and hot dogs. They are excessively full of calories, saturated fat, and artificial ingredients. It's my opinion that American meat, albeit delicious, is just too full of hormones. Many foreign governments prohibit its importation for that reason.

Rush Alternative: McDonald's Fish Sandwich, without the bread but with the cheese. (Don't be surprised; it's actually pretty good for you!)

Afternoon Snack (for those who must): A banana (sweet, tastes great, not too caloric, and easy to digest).

Dinner

Dieter's Trick: Eat as late as possible. Europeans think we're crazy eating dinner at five o'clock. Wait at least until seven, later if you can, then read the following suggestions in order to build a sensible menu.

Bouillon or consommé (not dry instant soup, which is too caloric)

Broiled or boiled chicken (don't eat the fatty skin) or broiled fish

Baked potato (with a bit of polyunsaturated margarine, but no sour cream, please)

Raw carrots, celery, and/or tomato slices

Glass of whole milk (8 ounces have 150 calories; an excellent source of Vitamin F)

Another Dieter's Trick: Save dessert until just before bedtime or *at least* until after the dishes. Then have a slice of cantaloupe, or a piece of pie or pound cake (if you can afford the calories), and one cup of coffee (black or with milk), unless it keeps you up at night.

I believe that anybody can take these simple dietary suggestions, along with a calorie counter, and rapidly become the master of his or her own figure. And while we're talking about eating, let's briefly discuss two other topics: fast foods and ethnic foods.

Fast Foods

Although they are not the basis of any sensible diet, fast foods are certainly part of the fabric of our life, and there are some good things to be said for them. For one thing, they won't hurt you. On the other hand, they tend to be excessively caloric, and they have also been said to cause acne. The acne connection is an unusual story, since it is the fast-food proprietor's desire for cleanliness that causes it. I mentioned earlier that iodides found in many vitamin and mineral supplement pills cause pustular reactions in the skin. These eruptions look just like big pimples. Many deep friers in the fast-food outlets are kept scrupulously clean by daily disinfecting with iodine. Inevitably, some of the iodine gets into the food itself, and it has been shown to cause pustular, acne-type eruptions.

But aside from that, fast foods constitute no health threat that I know of. If you're at Burger King or McDonald's, my advice is to choose the cheap burger. It's the lowest in weight, price, fat, and calories. And by the time you're back in the car, chances are you won't feel any less satisfied than if you had wolfed down the fatty and overstuffed deluxe version.

Better than the burgers are the fish sandwiches. And if you take off the bread, they're not even all that caloric. Burger King's Whaler and McDonald's Fish Sandwich are equally good; but skip the special sauce. As for the Colonel, it is a fact that chicken, even when it's deep-fried, is relatively low in calories. So skip the gravy and mashed potatoes, and enjoy the chicken with cole slaw instead.

Ethnic Foods

Again, remember that these are helpful hints; there's no intention here of exhaustively cataloging ethnic foods. I do want to recommend an excellent ethnic dish that's a true natural food and is available quite widely. It's called pizza! It's delicious, you can order it in small amounts, the crust is filled with B vitamins, and the cheese is a good source of Vitamin F. It's great, assuming you don't let it tip your calorie quota.

Chinese food, however, is the great fooler. With all those vegetables, it seems as though it must be good for you. But, personally, I don't think so. Chinese cooks fry everything in saturated fats, and tend to use too much monosodium glutamate (MSG). The dishes frequently contain shrimp and lobster, both of which contain heavy doses of acne-causing iodides. On the other hand, I love the taste of Chinese cooking, and have adjusted myself to the pitfalls by never ordering shellfish dishes and by asking the chef not to use MSG. He may or may not pay attention to me, but I do ask.

As for chopped chicken liver, which can hardly be considered Jewish anymore, it's a killer. Cholesterol is manufactured in the liver and hence quantities of it are found there. Eat liver in overabundance and you'll be setting yourself up for eruptive xanthoma (bumps of yellow fat that appear on the skin). Liver may also be acnegenic (many organ meats are), and because of its high cholesterol content when chopped and combined with mayonnaise, it might be cutting fifteen minutes off your life!

3

Fat Treatments and Cellulite

To begin with, cellulite rhymes with parakeet, not with neophyte. If you're among the legions mispronouncing it, take note. Next, since it is my own opinion that there is no such thing as 100 percent bunk, don't expect this chapter to be a hatchet job on the cellulite faddists. At least not completely.

There are two schools of thought on cellulite, one European and the other American. For overweight Europeans, the cellulite concept is very much in the mainstream of accepted thought on weight loss, and has been for many years. Most American doctors, as well as the medical societies and associations to which they belong, consider the cellulite boom nothing but a big hoax. However, Americans don't know everything. For years, this same American medical establishment collectively scoffed at acupuncture. Nowadays, acupuncture seems very credible and is available from licensed practitioners in major American cities.

Not surprisingly, the answer to the question "What is cellulite?" depends on whom you ask. Cellulite fanatics maintain that it is not the same as ordinary fat, that it resists ordinary diets and exercise and its removal requires a special and "new" approach. They point to skinny women with fatty thighs and say that these women could diet to death and still not get rid of the cellulite on their thighs. In order to differentiate cellulite from normal fat, they recommend squeezing the fatty area. If characteristic dimples are observed, it's the dreaded cellulite. I say this is nonsense.

If you were to make a biopsy of cellulite and put it under a microscope, you'd see the same big translucent cells you'd see in regular old fat. In fact, any piece of normal skin has fat cells, and the only potential problem with fat is a matter of degree. Skin is a series of layers, with the epidermis on top, the dermis below, and a layer of subcutaneous fat below that. Too much fat is unattractive, potentially unhealthful, and with rare exceptions a result of nothing more than eating too much. When a special chemical stain called Sudan Red is used to stain fat cells, both fat and cellulite appear identical. Even chemical analysis reveals no difference between our humble familiar fat and glamorous "new" cellulite. So, my personal approach to cellulite is that it is nothing more than an overabundance of normal fat. I do not believe that it is the result of any special metabolic problem, nor do I believe that it cannot be lost through diet restrictions and meaningful exercise.

Many years ago, in fact in my first weeks of private practice, I had as a patient a very rich, seventy-five-year-old Italian woman. She was quite stunning, in the way that rich older women sometimes are, and her looks were no accident. She had taken advantage of all the plastic surgery that money could buy, and was, in addition, a devotee of a practice I hadn't even heard of at the time. In my office, she extracted from her purse a vial filled with some enzyme preparation and set it on my desk.

"I owe my beauty to this," she said dramatically, pointing to the vial. Apparently, her doctor in Italy regularly injected her with enzymes and she wanted me to do the same. I remember this woman because she was my introduction to the European approach to injections. There are fewer restrictions on drugs in Europe than in the United States. Enzymes are rubbed on or injected into almost anyone. Moreover, you can even buy antibiotics over the counter at a pharmacy.

Sometimes cellulite therapy incorporates injections. Unfortunately, unpleasant side effects are rarely considered. Anyone who is or knows a diabetic is aware of the danger of insulin atrophy. The insulin enzyme that allows the diabetic to lead a normal life also destroys the fat in the tissues at the injection site. The skin there becomes yellowish and veiny, and the tissue collapses. This in itself seems convincing evidence that certain specific injections will cause fat to go away. But the problem is that no one as yet really knows how much of what to inject. You could wind up with dells in the place of your old bumps!

Still, as you read these words, there's little doubt that someone somewhere is getting an injection of chopped animal pancreas (or the like) for a cellulite problem. Even though there is no course of medication approved by the Federal Drug Administration (FDA), there are still doctors with both needles and willing patients. Some of these "doctors" are part of the vast netherworld of pseudomedical people who will inject anything and everything into anybody. Sometimes the injections are given alone, sometimes in conjunction with diet programs and exercise. Either way, I don't think much of them.

Fortunately, most cellulite practitioners aren't doctors, so they can't shoot you up with anything. An alternate approach used is to rub enzymes onto the skin, but I just don't see how this can work. The fat layer is way below the surface of the skin, and it's unlikely any rubbed-on enzyme could penetrate that deep. Many nondoctors have yet another gimmick, a process called "iontophorisis." The patient lies on a table (preferably in a dark room), has enzymes applied to the skin surface, then is given gentle electric shocks with small wires. This is not painful; in fact it can barely be felt. I don't think it actually does anything, but there are people who swear by these treatments and pay $10 to $20 per session. Sometimes in medicine improvements are attributed to the wrong causes. This may be a case in point.

Just as cellulite purports to be entirely different from

normal fat, cellulite faddists would have us believe that
it results from very specific things. They ascribe it to,
among other things, air pollution, poisonous foods, sed-
entary living, too few liquids—in short, the same things
that are bringing about the end of the world. I don't
favor air pollution, but I also don't see that it has much
to do with fat thighs. As for the dangerous edible pol-
luters of the human system, we find cellulite literature
warning us against things like pastrami, saltines, canned
soups, french fries, wine, bouillon cubes, and ketchup!
But it's long been known that eating too much rich food
will put on fat. The anticellulite diet is heavy on vegetables, fruit, cheeses, skim milk, and lots and lots of
water. But it is devoid of any new information. Every
dieter knows that lots of water and no rich food are the
usual regimen. The cellulite diets are conspicuously bare
of warnings against fruits that cause allergic reactions
(like the hives which so often show up after a large bowl
of strawberries) or the light foods (like iodide-rich shellfish and seaweed) that cause acne. What good is it to
have no fat on your thighs if it means having a face
full of pimples? Even more peculiar is the emphasis on
massage as part of a cellulite reduction program. While
massage feels wonderful, it certainly does not remove
fat.

There is no doubt that if you relax, get plenty of
exercise, and don't eat fatty foods, you'll look and feel
great. This is the essential message of the cellulite ex-
plosion. It's wonderful advice, but it's hardly news. It's
cheaper and ultimately much more valuable to look at
yourself honestly. Are bumpy thighs the only difference

between you and Raquel Welch? Will flat thighs make you into something you aren't now? Will they make people like you better? And if there is one specific roll or bulge of flabby tissue that's driving you crazy, have you considered plastic surgery? Despite the disdain so liberally heaped upon this procedure and the suggestion that it is only an indulgence of the vulgar nouveau riche, it happens to work very well. Plastic surgeons tuck tummies, bottoms—you name it—with terrific-looking results. What horrifies me is the thought of some quack shooting me up with heaven only knows what, prescribing an acnegenic diet, and charging an arm and a leg for pleasant but essentially useless massages.

My personal advice to those who think they have a cellulite problem is to relax and go on a diet. Chapter 2 is filled with useful suggestions on dieting. For now, I only want to caution you about certain things. First, go slow. Weight taken off too rapidly usually reappears just as fast. Don't take water pills, because they dehydrate the skin. And thyroid pills tend to thicken the skin. Beware of megavitamin treatments that can bring on bouts of acne and hormone treatments that might make your hair fall out. In short, slow, continuous dieting combined with regular exercise will take fat off anybody and is the healthiest reducing method.

For those of you who are too impatient for this advice, I wish you luck. Injections do work for some people; despite all their perils, they might work for you.

4

Sex and Your Skin

There is a definite correlation between a happy sex life and skin that's in good condition. The physiological basis of this is the strong effect sex hormones have on the skin. We're all actually highly sophisticated bio-feedback mechanisms, and our moods are directly related to hormone production.

The quaint notion that masturbation can cause hair to grow on the palms is funny, but the unsightly acne breakouts that sometimes plague already unhappy people are not amusing. It is generally true that happy people have good skin, while unhappy people often have skin problems. It's even more true that all existing skin conditions are aggravated by stress. Stress—and unhappiness—gang up on all of us from time to time, sometimes producing what's called a supratentorial problem (*supra*, meaning "above," and *tentorial*, referring to the tentorium, a part of the brain that separates the regions

23

devoted to involuntary and voluntary actions). Having this condition doesn't mean you're crazy, but it does mean that a disturbing life situation is causing brain signals to disrupt the delicate hormone balance of the body. Far too often, it's a tense or unfulfilling sex life that's at the bottom of it all. Putting that in order is beyond the scope of this book; suffice to say it's the unseen and unexpected cause behind many acne cases. (See Chapter 20 for a fuller explanation of hormones and acne.)

In addition to loving, fulfilling intercourse, many other sex matters are closely linked to good skin. About the most widespread of these is birth control pills, which are part of the sex life of many many millions of women. The Pill is essentially a hormone that fools the body into thinking it's pregnant. It's really a very clever idea, but each passing year the clamor against it grows. Many people are convinced the Pill ultimately induces cancer, heart attacks, and strokes. A considerable number of women simply refuse to take it. I can understand how they feel. Although the link is as yet unproven, the mere threat of cancer is frightening.

Birth control pills are essentially divided into two categories: estrogen-loaded pills and progesterone-loaded pills. It's really a trade-off between the two, but I vote for the estrogen in spite of the potential side effects, which may or may not include cancer, cysts, blood clots, or weight gain. I don't want to suggest that any of these conditions are inevitable if the estrogen-loaded pill is used. But some women do have adverse reactions. However, many more notice dramatic im-

provement in acne conditions after about three menstrual cycles. Menstruation can aggravate the herpes
virus (about which more later), but estrogen seems to
alleviate that also. What's more, estrogen often apparently retards hair loss (a big fear of menopausal
women) and smoothes the emotional side effects of
menopause. Sometimes the secret of those shockingly
sexy older women is estrogen.

On the other hand, the progesterone-loaded pills
have fewer side effects, and are considered relatively
safe. But progesterone's similarity to the hormone
androgen causes it to stimulate sebaceous oil glands on
the skin. The resulting excessive oiliness almost inevitably leads to pimples, especially when the progesterone
pills are imprudently prescribed for adolescents (up to
about age twenty-five). However, there are some women
on this type of pill who have no acne trouble at all,
although they are in the minority.

Are you suffering from some other side effects of the
Pill? Both types seem to encourage vaginitis and yeast
infections. Progesterone pills can contribute to hair loss.
What's worse (in the eyes of some), it can encourage
hair to grow on the face! Either pill might photosensitize you, bringing on a painful and unexpected sunburn
after only normal exposure. Then there's chloasma,
known as the "mask of pregnancy." This is a brownish
discoloration that appears on the upper cheeks of pregnant women. Remember, being on the Pill causes the
body to think it's pregnant.

In general, I believe a switch of birth control pills
(from the progesterone to the estrogen type) is a good

idea when acne won't respond to any other treatment. I also think more women should pay attention to what's in those pills they take practically every day so that they can be alerted to possible side effects. Ask your gynecologist what type he's given you. (Unfortunately, it's often impossible to tell by looking at the label.)

Besides stress related to intercourse and personal sexuality, stress is also related to anticipation: consider the "pimple before the big date." Here again the mind is interfering with normal hormonal activities of the body. Obviously, the prescription is to relax, but this is easier said than done. If you're getting married tomorrow afternoon, and have a pimple as big as the nose on your face, you'll want more help than soothing admonitions to calm down.

Fortunately, your dermatologist can help—with an "intralesional steroid injection." He takes a little needle and gives you a shot of an anti-inflammatory chemical right into the pimple. Amazingly, it really works. The pimple will disappear within twenty-four hours in almost every case. This is the fastest method; antibiotic pills or drying solutions applied topically won't have any effect the first day.

If a pimple isn't enough to send you to a doctor, you can take heart in the reminder that it always looks bigger to you than to the rest of the world. Try the following trick till it clears up. Apply calamine lotion first, then cover with makeup. I think the best makeup around is the medicated Liquimat line. Your pharmacist can custom-tint the stuff for you, whatever your skin color.

Under no circumstances should you cover acne eruptions with anything gooey or sticky like Vaseline.

To get your Liquimat custom-tinted you will have to
go to a good pharmacy. For nonesoteric things, the big
discount stores are fine. But for anything that requires
custom work, go to your local neighborhood pharmacy.
If you don't have any, ask your doctor to recommend
one. Don't expect discount prices. A really well-stocked
pharmacy has to charge more, both for the selection and
for the custom services it offers. At least it's tax deductible!

I want to cover one last major topic on the subject
of sex and skin—venereal disease. I'm sure you are aware
that we're in the middle of a modern VD epidemic.
But perhaps you are not familiar with the skin manifestations of such diseases. You might be interested to
learn that dermatology had its beginnings in the study
of syphilology, and dermatologists have traditionally
been consulted on venereal matters. Ironically, most
rashes in the genital area are *not* VD but usually fungal
or abrasion irritations. And the most common type of
VD—gonorrhea—has no skin manifestations at all. Gonorrhea is symptomized in women only by painful, malodorous greenish discharges. It's easy to cure with
massive doses of penicillin (shots, not pills), but it's just
as easy to become reinfected. Doctors call gonorrhea a
"Ping-Pong disease"—she gets it, infects him, he gets
it, and gives it back to her as soon as she's cured.

Other types of VD cause skin reactions. Syphilis, for
instance, is characterized in women by a painless sore,

usually on the labia. Sometimes the sore is hidden inside the vagina and, since it's painless, goes unnoticed. With or without therapy—consisting of large doses (shots, never pills) of penicillin—the sores go away after four to six weeks and everything seems fine. Anyone who doesn't go to a doctor during the primary phase of syphilis is just plain stupid. Usually about six weeks after the disappearance of the last sore, a generalized, ham-colored rash will spread over the body, concentrating on the palms and soles. This is usually accompanied by hair loss that results in a sort of moth-eaten look. Blood tests, which are sometimes negative in the primary stage, are always positive in the secondary stage of syphilis. Even more penicillin is needed to quash the disease at this point, but with or without treatment, the symptoms—but not the disease—will go away by themselves.

After the secondary stage, if untreated, syphilis can either lie dormant for a lifetime or it may eventually attack the brain, heart, and spinal cord, causing madness, blindness, and death. However, the disease is nothing to be afraid of: penicillin absolutely stops it dead. Some people foolishly take penicillin pills before or immediately after intercourse with syphilitics. These pills won't prevent infection, but they will mask the normal primary symptoms just enough either to fool you into thinking you don't really have it or to foul up the results of your blood test. So don't take them. If in doubt, the best protection against syphilis is to have your partner wear a condom. If you're really wondering, you should ask your partner if he has had any discharges (possibly gonorrhea) and examine him yourself for the telltale primary syphilitic sore.

Much more common nowadays, and certainly more talked about, is herpes simplex. Why it is called simplex is a mystery, since not very much is known about the herpes virus. There are two closely related types: type 1 causes those painful fever blisters some people get on the lips; type 2 causes a nearly identical painful blistering, except that it's normally on the genitals.

The hallmark of herpes is pain. Little multiple blisters will appear, and there's nothing to do except wait for them to run their course. There is a great debate as to how the virus is contracted in the first place. Some claim it's contagious and contractible during sex. Personally, I subscribe to the theory that the virus is contracted elsewhere, then waits deeply buried in nerve tissue until it is activated by a trauma of some sort. The trauma can be either a physical scrape or nick or a strong emotional reaction. However, even doctors are unsure, and everybody has a different opinion.

The worst part of herpes is that it has no cure. European physicians are trying out a vaccine that has not yet been approved by our Federal Drug Administration. No one claims it's 100 percent effective. Other experiments are being tried with treatments that employ sunlight, smallpox vaccine, and a variety of other drugs. But nothing as yet has been found that has the equivalent effect that penicillin has on syphilis.

If you suffer from herpes, you can give yourself some relief with cool compresses and medications such as Solarcaine, the sunburn preparation. In fact, almost any

OTC preparation that ends with "caine" will act as a mild local anesthetic. You might ask your druggist if he recommends a particular topical anesthetic for the condition.

There is one venereal disease that you actually can catch from a toilet seat. It is the result of an infestation of tiny mites and bears the appropriate-sounding name of scabies. Whether infection results from a dirty toilet or an infected sex partner, the symptoms are most uncomfortable. The little mites burrow down under the skin, literally set up housekeeping, and lay lots of eggs. The skin begins to itch maddeningly, and becomes covered with little reddened bumps. Affected areas most commonly include the genitals, wrists, and the skin lying between the fingers.

You won't be drummed out of the human race for catching a venereal disease, even one with a name like scabies. The worst treatment for VD is to keep it in the closet out of a misguided sense of shame. And if you have scabies, which many people do—there is practically an epidemic of it today—please remember that it is very easy to treat, although it is often misdiagnosed by an overworked doctor, who'll prescribe something for the itching and never discover the underlying cause. The proper treatment is with a prescription drug called Kwell. It comes in lotion and shampoo form, is left on for several hours, washed off, and applied again if needed. Since scabies are so highly contagious, both you and your sex partner must be treated.

Less common than scabies, but still a frequent problem, are venereal warts. They appear on the anal and genital regions and are caused by the same wart virus that raises them elsewhere on the body. If I described them as fungating and papilomitous, you probably wouldn't have a very clear idea of what they look like. So let me put it this way: If the same wart were on your hand, it would be a dry, roughly circular hardened lump. But in the moist genital areas, the lesion looks less distinct. It's also hard to treat, since the skin here is quite sensitive. Most doctors either burn the wart off or apply an organic compound called podophyllin, which creates a slow burning sensation about six to eight hours after application. At that point, you wash it off. The treatment is repeated in a few weeks' time if necessary. Podophyllin will cause the wart to dry up and eventually fall off.

Before I close this chapter, I want to mention one last venereal disease whose skin symptoms are very prominent. It's known as *molluscum contagiosum,* and it's caused by the largest known virus that attacks the human system. Molluscum has two highly distinctive features: It consists of *very* shiny bumps with depressed central dells, and it spreads like wildfire. To cure the condition, you must attack every single lesion. Fortunately this is simple to do. The virus is easily killed by disruption of the wartlike milieu in which it lives. So all the doctor has to do is to curette (scrape with a special small blade) each lesion quickly. That'll be enough to kill the virus and prevent its return. If the condition reappears immediately after treatment, it is because the doctor didn't get all the lesions.

In closing, here's a little venereal checklist for the morning you wake up with a sore on your genitals.

CHARACTERISTICS OF THE SORE	PROBABLE CAUSES
Firm and painless	Syphilis
Multiple, grouped, little blisters	Herpes
Little itchy red bumps	Scabies
Strangely symmetrical lesions	Almost always a bite, burn, or infected wound
Rapidly proliferating shiny bumps with central dells	Molluscum contagiosum
Nonitchy warty-looking lesions	Venereal warts

5

"Doctor, I Sweat All the Time!"

I hope none of the current advertising nonsense really convinces anyone that it's desirable to "stay dry." There's nothing wrong with perspiring. It's physiologically necessary for the elimination of excess heat and for the disposal of certain body wastes (such as urea, phosphates, and various other trace chemicals). And fresh perspiration on a clean body does not have an unpleasant odor.

Most people don't have any real problem coping with perspiration, and may prime-time television never dupe them into thinking they do! However, some people do sweat too much. What follows are the five most common sweat-related problems I see in my dermatology practice, together with simple advice on what to do.

Sweat Acne

This peculiar problem affects almost everybody from time to time. The archetype is the beautiful girl whose light summer blouse is hiding awful acne on her back and shoulders. Men, however, get it just as frequently. Ironically, it's much more common in people who don't have acne on the face. And it also gets worse in the summertime, when most acne improves.

Current thinking has it that hot weather and extra perspiration have a synergistic effect that stimulates excess sebaceous oil production on the skin. The result is greater incidence of occlusion (pores becoming clogged with oil), which in turn can lead to acne pimples. The solution is to dry up the area. Bathing with acne soaps, such as Fostex, SAStid, Acne-Aid, or Acnaveen, helps degrease the skin and strip away unwanted oil. Zeasorb Powder (one of my favorites) sprinkled on the affected area will soak up excess perspiration. It's also a good idea in hot weather to wear several layers of clothing. A cotton top underneath a woman's blouse, or an undershirt under a man's shirt, might seem illogical in the heat, but they soak up perspiration that might otherwise collect on the surface of the skin. And usually it's not that much hotter.

So here's a chance to do a little thinking yourself. Too often, there are professionals who will pump you full of antibiotics like tetracycline too fast. Maybe that acne on your back is due to nothing more than sweat.

Heat Rash

Also known as miliaria, this condition occurs when perspiration has no place to go. Sweat under occlusion, it's called, and you probably have encountered it on your back or buttocks while driving on a hot August day in the city or while playing tennis in a dress that's too tight. Tiny blisters form and the surrounding skin turns red and begins to itch. What happens is that you sweat so much that the sweat ducts become clogged. Little blisters will rise on the skin surface, or sometimes rupture under the skin, disseminating itchy, irritating sweat.

Heat rash particularly plagues soldiers in the tropics, but it can make life just as uncomfortable for career women in the office or homemakers in the suburbs. Wherever you are, if you have it, here's what to do: Dry it up. For most people, a lotion like calamine is all that's needed. But sometimes, when it's vividly red and particularly itchy, the best treatment is first to apply a steroid anti-inflammatory cream. You'll need a prescription for the cream, but it's nothing so exotic that your doctor won't know about. After the cream's applied, spread calamine over it. This will relieve the itching and at the same time promote drying. The calamine application also seems to encourage absorption of the soothing steroid cream. This treatment, incidentally, is an old trick whose effectiveness has dazzled many a patient.

Sweat Retention Syndrome

This is no doubt the worst and most common sweating problem. Young women are the most frequent, if not the only, sufferers, and it seems to bother people most in the wintertime. Why that should be, I don't know. However, I do believe sweat retention is closely related to stress.

When you sweat on the thighs for instance, you're probably just hot; when you sweat on the palms, you're usually nervous. Sweaty palms, in fact, are universally recognized as attributes of nervousness. The sweat retention syndrome is characterized by little sweat-filled blisters that erupt on the sides of the fingers and the sides of the feet. The blisters itch like crazy and most frequently occur on what I shall euphemistically call the finger of fate. Perhaps this bespeaks great body truths beyond the scope of this book.

The classic case is the woman who gets it just after the birth of a baby, just after a divorce, just before a bar exam, and so forth. So what can she do? The best treatment is probably to do nothing or perhaps take a Valium. If you can calm down without the Valium, so much the better. But in any event, emotional tranquility is going to help. Next, the temptation to overwash the hands à la Lady Macbeth must be resisted. This only irritates already irritated tissue, especially when a vigorous soapy washing is followed by application of a cream containing alcohol, notorious for aggravating rashes on eczematous people. Many supposedly soothing lotions and creams often contain things just as irritating.

If you must put something on, use plain old Vaseline, or maybe a little Aquacare. But the best idea is to wash the area once, leave it alone, and try to relax. Some people go on vacation to sunny climes and swear that sunshine clears up the blisters in double time. That may be, but perhaps the relaxation inherent in a vacation is what really speeds the healing.

The Sweating Palm

Risking redundancy, I say again that sweating palms are the hallmark of nervous people. But I know how embarrassing this problem can be, and I have several good solutions you can try for your damp hands while you devote other energies to achieving spiritual peace.

First a short diversion. The latest and in ways the strangest approach to this type of problem is through biofeedback. The goal of this method is to control whatever ails you by locating and altering the specific brain waves that cause it. This appeals to logic as a preferable alternative to chewing tranquilizers. But it's not yet very easy to find someone who can train you in biofeedback control. Some biofeedback centers do exist, usually in big hospitals, and more often than not they're engaged in research on high blood pressure. If the idea really captures your imagination, you can ask your internist if he knows a biofeedback center or perhaps just look around yourself. However, even if you locate one, they may not be willing to help with your sweating palms, but then again they might. (Beware of quacks.)

Much more accessible is a prescription for 25 percent aluminum chloride tincture. This you can easily obtain from your doctor and have filled just as easily by your local drugstore. What's even better, it is inexpensive. Twenty-five percent aluminum chloride tincture is a close chemical relative of the aluminum chloride salts contained in all the big brand-name deodorants. It is thought to change the electrical polarity of the sweat glands, thereby halting perspiration flow to the surface. It really does work well, and lasts a long time. Short of a prescription for the 25 percent tincture, you can always apply underarm spray deodorant directly to the palms.

A stronger approach would be to tan the hands the way leather is tanned. For this, soak the palms in a tanning agent. A good one is tannic acid, which you probably already have in your kitchen cabinet in the form of teabags. You can brew a large cup of tea with three or four bags, let the water cool a bit, then soak your hands daily for about five minutes. Gradually, you'll see thicker palms, and less sweat.

Or, you can mix Zeasorb Powder with what's called 20 percent fluffy tannic acid. Actually, your pharmacist has to do it for you, since fluffy tannic acid is a prescription item. It's also something of a pain in the neck to make this prescription up, so expect him to charge you accordingly. The combination, however, is very effective when all else fails.

The Malodorous Armpit

Brome hydrosis is the scientific name for smelly sweat. When fresh from the sweat gland, perspiration does not smell bad. However, skin bacteria soon get to work on it, and the by-products of bacterial metabolism can be very offensive. Instead of tackling the sweat, you'll have better luck attacking the bacteria. Changing the flora of the skin surface will inevitably alter the smell of your perspiration.

This is exactly the opposite approach of brand-name deodorants. They attempt to stop perspiration, or at least severely curtail it. Some years back, one of the large drug companies introduced a Vitamin E deodorant that had an interesting concept behind it. Vitamin E is a known antioxidant, and its presence on the skin tended to hinder bacterial oxidation. But so many people became sensitized to Vitamin E by this product that it provoked allergic responses all over the place. It was finally withdrawn from the market.

Unfortunately, the subject of body odor is furtively treated by most people. But if you have it, I advise you to attack the skin bacteria with deodorant soap containing antibacterial agents. Dial, Safeguard, Palmolive Gold, and so on are all just fine. Just one caution: These soaps can make you disposed to a bad sunburn (photosensitization).

If you need something stronger, you can ask your doctor to prescribe pHisoHex. This used to be an over-the-counter item, until the hexachlorophine it contains was linked to brain damage in infants. But soaking a newborn child in hexachlorophine is hardly the same as washing your adult armpits or groin area with pHisoHex. The stuff happens to be a superior sterilizer with extraordinary staying power that discourages bacterial reestablishment.

Before ending this chapter, there is one final topic to discuss. Did you know that the sweat of a rhinocerous is red? It's called *chrome hydrosis,* meaning colored perspiration. And not only rhinos but perfectly nice people occasionally suffer from it too! Not very much is understood about this, but the condition is generally acknowledged not to be dangerous. If you have it, I don't know what to tell you, except that you need not be terribly worried. It's not fatal, but neither is it curable at present.

6

The Art
of Using Makeup

There are two major schools of thought on the subject
of makeup. One would have us believe that it's utterly
without value, and in fact harmful. They claim makeup
clogs the pores and may contain coal tars, both of
which lead to acne. And it is true that the incidence of
cosmetic-related acne has become so great in recent years
that medical parlance contains a new term—"acne cosmetica."

The other school maintains, with substantial justifi-
cation, that cosmetics are attractive and actually protect
the face from the dirt and grime of daily living. And
there are no lack of mature women, sometimes well into
their fifties or even older, with beautiful complexions.

These women have always used makeup, and they are living testimonials to its benefits.

As for myself, I've become something of a convert to the use of makeup in the last year, at least as long as it's used intelligently.

This isn't easy, particularly if you read the women's magazines. Let me say right here that I am a fan of the women's magazines and think they are a source of terrific information. But they often contain confusing and contradictory advice when it comes to cosmetics. Confusion, however, is the gist of the cosmetics industry.

Successfully applied, cosmetics even out your complexion and artistically highlight (or understate) your features. I'm all for experimenting with makeup, but be sure to build around your own natural endowments. If your face just isn't suited to a current makeup trend or fashion, it's an unfashionable mistake to make yourself up that way. The girls on the covers of *Vogue* are beautiful, but one tends to forget that it takes hours to make them up. Not to mention that noses and cheekbones like theirs are not exactly standard equipment.

In my opinion, good makeup makes the complexion look smooth without clogging the pores, enhances the best points of the facial structure, and is not unduly affected by the whims of passing fashion. Fortunately, fashion passes quickly, so we can hope that the bruised cheekbone look will be back in hibernation by the time you read this.

To intelligently choose appropriate makeup products, you must first determine whether your skin is oily or dry. For this, I refer you to the skin test in Chapter 13. In general, young women tend to have oily skin, which gradually dries up as the years progress. The skin of the more mature woman is typically much drier than that of her younger sisters and can tolerate oil-based products much better. So a product that has ideally suited an older woman for years might very well give her daughter a bad case of acne.

In the pages that follow, I'm going to discuss the basic component stages of makeup from the point of view of both acne-prone and oil-starved skin. It shouldn't be hard to fit yourself into the range of suggestions below. Your goal is to construct your own minimal makeup kit, which will be neither expensive, nor acnegenic, nor time-consuming to use.

Cleansing

The function of a good cleanser is to remove all the soot, grease, dirt, old makeup, and oil from your face without harming the skin. Most younger women need nothing more exotic than a bar of soap. Ivory or plain Palmolive (not the Gold deodorant variety) are just fine. For skin that tends to be a bit oily, I like Neutrogena, which is very pure, practically transparent, and has a slightly drying effect.

Many young women still must contend with acne problems, and for them I would recommend one of the acne soaps. Don't be dissuaded because you think they're only for kids or will somehow damage your complexion. That's nonsense. Your acne is very likely the result of excessive oil secretion, and the best thing you can do is to dry up the oil as much as possible. Fostex is a very good antiacne drying soap, as are SAStid, Sulphur Soap, and Acne-Aid. These are all available in drugstores. Again, don't worry about bruising your tender skin—they're good for you!

If you're really having trouble with acne and have terribly oily skin, then use one of the soaps containing little granules, such as Pernox or Ionax. You can get these also at the drugstore, and they're great for really deep cleansing of the face.

Older women with dryer skin can use much milder cleansers. For them, cold cream is the best. Of all the cold creams, I prefer Ponds. It's a basic cold cream, essentially nothing more than glycerine and rosewater, and it costs under a dollar. If you like washing with soap, then I recommend a cold-cream soap like Dove, which has a time-tested formula and is very mild and safe, or one of the superfatted soaps like Alpha Keri Soap or Lowila Cake. I know "superfatted" doesn't sound so great, but the soaps themselves are pleasant smelling, very nice to use, and excellent for oil-starved skin.

Cleanse your face first thing every morning, whether you're young or old. If you substantially change or reapply makeup at any time during the day, cleanse the face and start from scratch. Clean all your makeup off before you go to bed. One final caution about cleansing: Don't use hot water. Hot water causes vasodilation, an expansion of the capillaries in the skin. This has a cumulative effect over the years and can lead eventually to redness, blotchiness, and obvious veins. So, *always* wash your face with cool or lukewarm water.

Moisturizers and Foundations

Some women need to apply both a moisturizer and a foundation, some women need neither, and some women need only one or the other. It depends on how dry or oily your skin is and on the evenness of your complexion tone. It's very possible that you don't need a moisturizer at all, and it is just as possible that an ordinary moisturizer will perform the work of a foundation for you.

Foundation makeup has two functions: It smoothes over and fills out imperfections; and it provides a background and anchor for the makeup to follow. As a matter of fact, blushers and powders, and so forth wouldn't even stay on the skin without a foundation. It's rather like spackling and priming a wall before painting, albeit with a (hopefully) lighter touch.

The goal of this step in the makeup process is to obtain a smooth, velvety surface that hydrates the skin without clogging the pores. Avoiding occlusion (pore clogging) is particularly important for younger women, whose skin is naturally more oily than that of older women. Aquacare and Carmol, which contain urea, are excellent products for young women. Urea is an aquaphilic substance that chemically attracts and holds the skin's natural moisture without being oily or occlusive. Also good are Clinique Makeup Base and Revlon's Charlie Matte Base, both good hydrators and nonoily.

Plenty of other products are equally good, but the point here is to illustrate the importance of nonoiliness for young women.

For really bad skin, I recommend Liquimat. This foundation has medicine in it (primarily sulphur and alcohol) that combats acne-causing oiliness, and it comes in ten different shades. What's more, it's inexpensive and covers especially well.

Older women with typically drier skin want different things from a foundation. They need moisture, and their skin can more easily tolerate oil-based products. It's generally true that the older you get, the more cosmetic products you can use without side effects. I'm personally a fan of Elizabeth Arden's Everyday Moisture line. I think Estee Lauder makes a good product too, as do quite a number of other manufacturers. You can go whole hog, if you like, and indulge in mink oils and musk oils, or pay $25 for Geminesse's Cream Hydracel. There is a lot of latitude in experimentation with moisturizers. Of course, all these things do approximately the same thing as Crisco, but not many women really care to rub Crisco on their faces.

Finishing Touches

Having laid a good foundation, the palette is yours, and any artfully applied color will look good so long as it complements your natural coloring. Liners, powders, rouges, pots of this and that, are all so carefully tested by their manufacturers that there is little chance of any of them causing you any harm. I don't see much point in paying more for hypoallergenic preparations either. The additional protection they provide is so minimal as not to be worth the extra price.

Your ultimate look depends on your mood and on a lot of personal experimentation. You can make yourself look distinguished, coquettish, glamorous, or whatever by varying colors and brush strokes. Now, having said that nearly any makeup line will do, I feel inclined to mention Clinique and Mary Quant, which are both nonacnegenic and have tremendous variety. I'll also give you a tip, if you don't already know, about Bonne Bell Snow Tan, which is great. It gives you a Puerto Rican tan in the middle of winter, and will fool anyone.

As far as eye makeup goes, anything goes. Lots of women get rashes around the eyes, but the overwhelming cause is nail polish! This happens when the eyelashes are flicked with not-quite-dry fingernails.

Addenda

Some miscellaneous items come to mind, which I want to discuss before going on to other things. The first is astringents, those strong-smelling, alcohol-based liquids whose purpose is to degrease very oily skin. Manufacturers often call them "clarifying lotions," and they're recommended in addition to cleansers for oily-skinned people who don't use much makeup. Astringents tend to plump up the pores and make them look temporarily smaller. Georgette Klinger makes a superb clarifying lotion, as do Revlon and Estee Lauder. Seba-Nil is another good one, especially for acne-prone women. And of course, plain old witch hazel does the job exceedingly well—and for the least money. After-shave lotions are essentially astringents, and as such are the best makeup for men.

Facial masks, as I pointed out in Chapter 1, have been with us since ancient times and have made something of a comeback recently. My feeling is that they make you feel good and do absolutely no harm. Just don't expect a mask that you buy in the drugstore to take years off your appearance. It won't. But it will deep-cleanse the face, promote some minimal peeling, and tighten up the pores—at least temporarily. You might try some of the recipes in Chapter 1 for organic masks you can make at home. Or you can shop around and try the various masks on the market. The prime criterion for a good facial mask is whether it feels good and is pleasant to use. The mechanics of applying it seldom vary, which is to say that you mix it up, paint it on, let dry for ten minutes or so, then wash off with water. The only one worth specific mention here is the Seba-Nil Mask, undoubtedly *the* mask for acne sufferers or very oily-skinned people.

Complexion lotions are preparations designed to cover acne trouble spots. They are not meant to be spread over the entire face but only over bad pimples. Clearasil Lotion is excellent, so just because you're not a teenybopper, don't rule it out. Propa-PH is good too, as are Fostex Lotion and Sulfacet Lotion. Elizabeth Arden's Medicated Lotion is a little fancier and also does the job well. Which is to say that it covers up the pimple without irritating or making it worse.

Finally there are emollients, whose presence in makeup is often advertised by cosmetic manufacturers. An emollient is a substance halfway between a cream and an ointment. That means it has properties that lie between the quick-vanishing, nonoily creams and the long-lasting, sometimes acnegenic ointments, and has the benefits and side effects of both.

7

Cosmetic Surgery

Cosmetic surgery is elective. It's not imperative to health; you'll live the same number of years without it; and it's not tax deductible. But on the other hand, life is short, and happiness is at a premium. That thought is really what's at the bottom of my predisposition to cosmetic surgery. I approve wholeheartedly of the pursuit of happiness.

But operations are nothing to take lightly. Surgery is surgery, and every operation has its element of risk. Beware of the doctor who intentionally makes light of a cosmetic operation. There is no such thing as a procedure that is painless, causes no disruption in your life, and results in a perfect transformation. Cosmetic surgery won't make an unhappy person into a happy one. If no one wants to go out with you, it's probably because of your personality, not your pockmarks. Expect improvement, not perfection. But there will always be people whose expectations are unrealistic and whose egos aren't strong enough to bear continued unpopularity. Some postcosmetic surgery patients actually commit suicide.

Notwithstanding the drawbacks, I think cosmetic surgery can work wonders for many people. Perhaps you're wondering how you would choose a doctor if you really have decided to go through with it.

For one thing, all the people who perform plastic surgery aren't necessarily plastic surgeons. A doctor is licensed to perform any medical procedure, and you'll find plenty of nose alterations done by ear/nose/throat specialists, and plenty of eye-debagging (officially called blepharoplasty) performed by opthomologists. If you are looking for a good plastic surgeon get one who specializes in the procedure you are interested in (face-lifts, noses, eyes, and so forth), and be sure that he is "board certified."

Your public library has the *Directory of Medical Specialists*. This publication lists all the doctors who are certified for competency by a variety of specialty boards that sit under the auspices of the American Medical Association. There's a board for every specialty—dermatology, plastic surgery, internal medicine, and so forth. Applicants undergo thorough oral and written examinations in order to be board certified because certification by the various American boards is an internationally recognized demonstration of merit. You shouldn't be afraid to ask any doctor if he's board certified. Chances are, you'll be able to see his framed certificate from the "American Board of (whatever his specialty)" right on the wall—look for it always.

There are, however, some older doctors who are absolutely brilliant in their fields but who aren't board certified. Usually, there's a good reason that has something to do with being a struggling doctor during the Depression and not having had the money to pay the board fees. Many of these stories are absolutely valid. But my personal opinion is that any *young* doctor worth his salt is certified. If he isn't, he's not the best available.

Financial arrangements should be discussed as openly as possible. For one thing, it is customary to pay for a cosmetic operation before it is performed. This seems to fly in the face of all the political consumerism we're pumped full of these days. But the reason for this tradition is the tendency of some patients to find fault with an operation after it's performed, then to seize upon the imagined fault as an excuse not to pay the bill. If you can't pay the whole amount on the day of surgery, you should discuss it frankly with the doctor. Some doctors take credit cards; some will allow you to make payments in stages. Know what's expected of you, and be sure your arrangements are clear.

The price for any given cosmetic procedure will vary significantly from city to city, and from doctor to doctor. These operations are expensive, usually costing in the thousands of dollars. It is possible to find board-certified doctors in foreign countries who can do an excellent job for a relatively low price. Some people go to places like Brazil and figure that their air fare added to the reduced doctor's fee down there will equal the cost of the operation at home. Trips like this also provide the opportunity to drop completely out of sight for the weeks when you're black and blue and to have a vacation. Here at home, the doctor in the suburban town will sometimes do the job more cheaply than the doctor on Park Avenue in Manhattan. But wherever you look, remember to look for a doctor who does *lots* of whatever it is you want done.

What follows are some of the most commonly sought elective cosmetic procedures, together with a short discussion on the ins and outs of each.

Face-Lift

The results can be really beautiful. A good doctor can do equally effective lifts of the breasts, buttocks, and thighs, using essentially the same procedure as on the face.

The typical face-lift patient is over forty, either male or female, and suffers from accumulated wrinkles and sagging flesh. Face-lifting (or any other kind of lifting) does not affect the muscles at all. The doctor makes easy-to-hide incisions in the skin, then undermines the skin tissue with a scalpel, pulls it back to restore tautness, and finally snips off the extra skin. The scars are put in invisible places behind the ears or under the hairline. The face looks tighter, more youthful, and the sags are eliminated. There's considerable black and blue from bleeding under the skin, but that usually goes away in a few weeks.

However, as years pass, the skin will continue to sag so that in about five years you may want another lift. Fortunately, the same procedure can be repeated, but it does get harder each time.

Face-lifts provide a good opportunity to do eyes, nose, and so forth at the same time. Having several procedures at once is less costly than undertaking the operations separately. Because of the cost and the trauma involved, you'd better be as prosperous as you are healthy.

Blepharoplasty

This operation gets rid of droopy eyelids and baggy circles under the eyes. With this nice, short, very effective procedure, the surgeon makes an incision along the natural lines around the eye, then snips out the little pockets of fat beneath the skin. It can be done in the doctor's office, and about the only thing he need be particularly cautious about is not to take out too much. If he does, you may have trouble closing the eye—or even become blind. Fortunately, this rarely happens, especially when you're dealing with someone who does lots of eyes.

Prices for any of these operations vary so considerably that I have not even attempted to quote figures. Blepharoplasty, for instance, can cost from $250 to $2,500, which I know is not a helpful answer. Just remember that prices (and malpractice insurance rates) go only one way.

Hair Transplants

Not only men lose their hair. Women have just as much trouble. The ideal candidate for hair transplanting is over thirty and has well-demarcated areas of baldness. Diffusely thinning hair is not well suited for transplants, as the following description of the procedure will show.

An instrument called a hair transplant punch is used almost like a cookie cutter to take out circular chunks 3½ millimeters in diameter from areas of thick hair on your scalp (usually at the back). These "plugs," as they're called, are then fitted into identical-sized holes that have been prepared on the bald area. It's an ongoing process that requires commitment from the patient, who must be prepared to keep coming back for months or even years. Hundreds or thousands of plugs may ultimately be transplanted, and they can't all be done at once. Each plug contains healthy hair follicles that require time to root. The trauma of the transplant may cause the hair to fall out initially, but it grows back within sixty days. The plug blends with the surrounding skin into which it has been transplanted.

Despite the cost ($5 to $20 per plug), and the lengthy follow-up period, transplants are very effective. The technique isn't hard, but you'll get the best results from a doctor who's had lots of practice. There's an art to good-looking transplants that comes only from experience. Oftentimes, the best transplants are done by dermatologists.

Mammary Augmentation and Reduction

First we'll deal with mammary augmentation, or breast enlargement. It's another very safe and simple procedure, although it does require hospitalization. The breast is lifted up and an incision is made along the bottom where the scar won't be seen. The doctor then makes a little pocket, into which he inserts a bag filled with silicone. Then he sews you back up, and you're ready to go topless!

There was a time when these operations were done with injections of free silicone, but silicone's tendency to float around the body resulted in the invention of the bagged variety. Although your breasts will look completely normal, you'll always be able to feel the silicone bag with your hands.

Mammary reduction consists of surgical removal of excess breast tissue. In cases of oversized, sagging, or painful breasts, the doctor will make the incision below or on the side of the breast, remove the excess, snip off the extra skin, and resew the incision. The procedure is fairly major, but the cosmetic effect is usually very successful.

Procedures for Acne Scarring

Many of us bear disfiguring scars from prolonged battles with adolescent acne. Once the acne is finally burnt out, there are many things that can be done.

You've probably heard of people who've had their

faces sanded. The correct term for this is "dermabrasion." A plastic surgeon or dermatologist spot-freezes the skin with an aerosol freeze spray, then literally grinds it down with a dermabrader. These tools have diamond burrs that remove frozen flesh quickly. The procedure is usually recommended for cases of particularly deep scarring. Even so, dermabrasion has serious drawbacks: it hurts; you bleed profusely; and the dermabrader is hard to control even by the most experienced hands. Sometimes scarring results on top of the acne scars that were supposed to be removed. Sometimes the skin lightens or darkens inexplicably.

I much prefer a procedure called "chemabrasion." This process is often called face "peeling," which is exactly what it is. The dermatologist paints the face with a strong chemical (like trichloroacetic acid) that actually burns off the top layers of skin. Usually the chemical application is repeated twice, and after each session the patient returns home to wait for the skin to peel. Chemabrasion makes scars and pits shallower and induces a natural swelling that tends to pop the scars out a bit. It's much less painful and much less expensive than dermabrasion. It's also good for getting rid of fine lines and wrinkles.

It's possible to plump out very deep, individual scars in much the same way your breasts are plumped out—with silicone. At this writing, the Federal Drug Administration is not 100 percent convinced about silicone.

At present only ten doctors in the country are licensed, under "experimental drug" licenses, to practice this type of silicone therapy, which works as follows. The doctor undermines the scar with a needle and simply shoots the silicone into the skin until it's pumped up to an even surface. By the time you read this, the government may have approved the treatment. In the meantime, you can write to the FDA and request their list of doctors if the idea intrigues you sufficiently. Be careful: this treatment is rumored to be widely available from unlicensed practitioners.

Besides, there's an approved (albeit expensive) alternative that utilizes the body's own blood. It's called "fibrin foam," and a small group—patients of the originator—has been getting the treatment for years. Only with a recent posthumous article in the medical press has fibrin foam suddenly come into vogue.

Fibrin is a chemical by-product of your blood clots and is part of every scar that forms on your body. It's expensive and complicated but possible to separate the fibrin from a sample of your blood. Of course, your doctor has to have the facilities to do this. The biggest advantage of fibrin is that it already belongs to the rest of your body, which almost entirely precludes rejection, migration, or allergic reaction.

The same deep individual scars or pits that lend themselves to silicone treatments also are good candidates for fibrin foam. The doctor will undermine the skin at the bottom of the scar and pump in the fibrin until the affected area plumps out to everybody's satisfaction. It's a very good procedure but not as yet widely available.

Cryosurgery

Older people have acne behind them, but they have a new set of problems to face. A lifetime's worth of excessive sun exposure often causes skin cancers (which incidentally are not particularly dangerous and certainly not life-threatening), sun spots, and raised, scaly keratoses. Cryosurgery does not involve the use of knives or needles; rather, an application of liquid nitrogen spot-freezes each lesion. The cryosurgical apparatus has a point that is touched to the lesion, causing a blister to rise. In the process of healing, the lesion itself will fall off, to be replaced by new skin.

Electronic Facial

Also for older folks' problems, the electronic facial is cheaper than cryosurgery and often works just as well. Like cryosurgery, this technique is the province of a dermatologist. He uses an electric needle to go over the face briefly touching each bad area. These might include sun spots, obvious veins, wrinkles, and those scaly age spots we call keratoses. It hurts a little, and causes a mild irritation and production of edema fluid by the traumatized skin. Shortly after a treatment, the lesions will fall off and be replaced by fresh healing skin. The edema fluid will tend to plump out wrinkles temporarily, for a month or so. Swollen or otherwise obvious veins are literally fried by the electric current. They die, dissolve, and are absorbed by the system.

I recommend the process wholeheartedly for the typical problems of older skin. A final tip: The imaginary overworked doctor who, for the purposes of illustration, prescribes the wrong thing throughout this book may see redness and prescribe an anti-inflammatory steroid cream. However, if the redness stems from surfacing veins, steroid creams will make the condition *worse*.

8

The New Skin Machines and Other Skin Care Aids

While technology continues to encroach on our private lives, the most exciting news in skin care is decidedly naturalistic. What's more, it's bound to make many an old wife—and mother—smile with the satisfaction of having been right all along.

I refer to epiabrasion, a hot new concept that holds out the promise of better-looking skin to both young and old. Epiabrasion boils down to little more than scrubbing your face for a prolonged period every morning. The only reason this idea can possibly be considered "new" is that it goes against the accumulated advice of cosmetologists, dermatologists, and sundry manufacturers, who for years have been telling women to gently pat on all manner of expensive preparations. It now looks as if they should have been telling them to scrub their faces instead!

Regular epiabrasion takes off a few layers of cells every morning. It helps young and extra-oily skin combat acne because it keeps the face extra clean and oil-free as it scrapes away incipient oil plugs that might otherwise cause pimples. Average normal skin acquires an attractive glow that comes from cleanliness, good circulation, and a good cell-turnover rate. Regular epiabrasion results in plumper skin cells that are better organized. This temporary plumping tends to smooth out fine lines and wrinkles too. The sun-damaged skin of older people responds just as well. Scaly and reddened areas become clearer, cleaner, and better looking. The process removes crusty keratoses and stimulates the growth of fresh new skin.

In fact, there have been studies with a scanning electron microscope that clearly show skin cells to be in better condition after regular epiabrasion. These studies were conducted by the 3M Company, the manufacturer of my favorite epiabrasion product, the Buf-Puf. You can buy a Buf-Puf very reasonably at most drugstores, either as part of an acne kit, complete with special drying soap, or all by itself. It's a circular synthetic pad that lasts about a month. Although more abrasive than a washcloth, it's not painful. It is also cheap, does not require a prescription, and is backed with scientific evidence that it really works.

Bear in mind that you can do almost as well with

organic products like Tawashi or loofah, or your own washcloth for that matter, which all utilize the same epiabrasion concept. However, my favorite is still the Buf-Puf, because of its uniformity of texture and its convenient size and shape.

The epiabrasion regimen is simple. Take your Buf-Puf (or whatever) and scrub the face for about a minute each morning. Be careful not to overdo it. Within two to three weeks, you should have increased the morning scrub to about three minutes' duration. And if other areas of the body are giving you problems—for instance, acne on the shoulders—then use the Buf-Puf there too.

If your skin becomes irritated, stop. Perhaps you'll be able to start again in a few days, weeks, or even months, although there are some people with sensitive skin who won't be able to tolerate epiabrasion.

If you have normal skin, then you can epiabrade with plain old soap. Any brand you like is fine. If you have an oil or acne problem, use an acne soap or a drying soap like Neutrogena. If you're older or have dry skin, then combine the Buf-Puf with a superfatted soap like Aveeno Bar, Lowila Cake, Oilatum, or one of the more commercial brands that contain oil or cold cream like Dove or Caress. Whatever your skin type, you will note a definite improvement, usually in two to three weeks. Don't stop, though; keep it up regularly, and make it part of your daily regimen. It will make you look better and even keep away acne.

Now to the machines. Undeniably the best one for your skin is the sunlamp. It gives you an attractive tan, and promotes a mild peeling that's very helpful for acne, eczema, psoriasis, and even dandruff. To the best of my knowledge, there has never been a reported case of skin cancer due to a sunlamp. But the apparatus should be used with caution, as it can damage unprotected eyes, or give you a severe sunburn.

You can buy a sunlamp in a drugstore, but don't get a heatlamp by mistake. General Electric, Sperti, and Norelco are a few of the big manufacturers. The light rays are all the same, but prices depend on the various stands, goggles, and reflectors that may or may not be part of the package. The only thing you really need besides the lamp is a pair of goggles. Under no circumstances should you use a lamp without them. Sunglasses aren't good enough; the goggles must be opaque.

Your first time under the sunlamp should be for no more than five seconds. Stay under for an additional five seconds for each successive day, until you have a nice golden color. That should happen when you hit three to four minutes. Then stay under the lamp for that length of time every day to maintain your color. Like epiabrasion, the sunlamp should become a part of your daily routine. It's particularly not something to start, stop, and start again, because to do so can provoke an acne flare. Each time your skin is under the lamp, it tends to thicken somewhat. There is a corresponding tendency for skin to get a bit thinner without exposure to the lamp. This back-and-forth effect can sometimes clog pores and lead to the same kind of pimples that occasionally hit northeners on a southern beach vacation.

If you start to burn before your daily dosage hits

two to three minutes, then naturally you should decrease the dosage or postpone the next five-second increase for a few days. For a darker tan, stay under longer than three minutes daily. Whatever you do, do it every day, do it gradually, protect your eyes, and you'll be quite safe. If you notice a little wrinkling, don't be frightened. It's only pseudo-wrinkling, a temporary condition caused by dehydration from the sunlamp. Apply some Aquacare, a nonoily cream that naturally attracts and holds moisture in the skin. Carmol is a stronger version of Aquacare.

Another very simple skin device is a small metal instrument that looks at first glance as if it belongs in a dentist's office. It's called a comedo extractor (comedo is the official term for pimples or blackheads).

I think this device is very good because I believe that pimples and blackheads should be squeezed out. But there are two dangers in squeezing: botching the job and making the pimple even bigger, or botching the job in the "triangle of death." This ominously titled zone lies not off the coast of Bermuda but right on your own face, on either side of your nose, and on the forehead area between your eyes. It's called the triangle of death because a bad infection here can drain into a section of the brain where a subsequent infection can be fatal. Now I know every one of you has had pimples in this area, has squeezed a few of them quite badly, but you're still alive and reading this page. Well, you were just lucky. The fact that nearly everyone is similarly lucky does not negate the possibility of contracting a fatal infection. They're not that rare, either.

The comedo extractor has a point at one end, and what looks rather like a miniature spoon with a hole in it at the other. It usually costs $2 to $5 at a good drugstore. The technique for squeezing pimples and blackheads is easy but requires a bit of practice to perfect. Briefly, you use the pointed end to nick the side of a pimple, or deroof a blackhead. Then you center the hole at the other end of the extractor over your nick and press carefully from the side. You'll get the hang of it quite quickly, but remember not to nick or press too vigorously. You might want to practice your technique on the black spots on a grapefruit or an orange. Don't laugh. Doctors practice all sorts of things —like dermabrasion and injections—on oranges.

One of the most widely known skin machines is the electric needle used by the professional who practices electrolysis. This is the famous method of hair removal that might soon be going into eclipse, but more about that later.

Unfortunately, electrolysis hurts. The needle is inserted into each hair follicle, the juice is turned on, and ouch! This fries the hair root and allows the unwanted hair to be plucked out, hopefully never to appear again. Of course, the method, like all methods, is not 100 percent effective, so a certain number of those hairs are going to grow back again. Many sittings are usually required, since the patient can stand only just so much pain. It's the electric current that really hurts, but the needle doesn't feel so great either. Interestingly, electrolysis is the popular method of choice for removing little veins from the face. Again, the needle is inserted and the electric current fries the vein, which is then absorbed by the surrounding tissue.

There is also a do-it-yourself item called a Perma-Tweez, which is available through mail-order ads in many of the women's magazines. Perma-Tweez looks rather like a ballpoint pen. You insert the point into the follicle, then press the button to fry your hair root. Some women swear by Perma-Tweez, but sometimes it can be pretty uncomfortable.

But what of all the advertisements for "painless" hair removal? Now we come to Depilatron, a franchise operation that utilizes ultrasonic waves to fry hair roots in much the same way that microwave ovens cook food. I think it's worlds better than conventional electrolysis primarily because it is absolutely painless. It is also extremely safe, somewhat more effective since fewer hairs return, and faster since many more hairs can be removed in a sitting because of the lack of discomfort.

Depilatron franchises advertise in local magazines and newspapers and are often found in good department stores. You'll be treated by a trained professional who zaps each follicle with a stylus attached to a patented Depilatron box with a foot pedal to regulate the ultrasonic waves. You'll neither hear nor feel a thing. There's no question that this is the preferred method for removal of unwanted hair.

Back in the do-it-yourself department is an apparatus called The Skin Machine. This is a $10 to $14 or so item, made and patented by Clairol and available at drug and department stores. It's a box with a small rotating brush that supposedly deep-cleans and stimulates the face. It's actually rather good for acne problems when used in combination with one of the granulated soaps like Pernox or Komex. But the bristles tend to be soft, and you can do the same thing with your own washcloth, or better yet with the aforementioned Buf-Puf.

Finally we come to facial saunas, which are also the subject of some debate. Essentially, a facial sauna is a plastic cup with rubberized sides that covers the entire face. Sunbeam, Norelco, and a number of other manufacturers make them. The steam makes some people feel good, and steam-softening the skin will open the pores and make blackhead or pimple extraction easier. On the other hand, steam seems somehow to irritate the pores of acne-prone people. Some maintain that these saunas actually induce acne flares, while others report that their acne is helped. So, whom do you believe? Try it yourself if the concept appeals to you and see what happens.

Older people typically find these steam saunas to their liking. If you're older and you'd like to try an easy steam regimen, after the sauna wash your face with Oilatum or any of the superfatted soaps. Then paint on a mask of nothing but egg whites. After the mask, pat the face with warm water, and apply your favorite moisturizer. The cleansing action the steam and the Oilatum combined with the slight peeling from the mask will make you look and feel temporarily much better.

9

How to Take a Bath

So you think you know how already! Joking aside, most of you probably do. However, the bathing habits of dry-skinned people typically make dry skin worse. And acne-prone people usually overlook opportunities during the daily bath or shower to help their skin.

It's an established fact that bathing dries the skin. I know that on the surface this seems to go against common sense. Nonetheless, skin that has been soaked in water and allowed to dry will manifest symptoms of dehydration. The way the typical oil-based moisturizer works is to seal pores shut and lock in existing moisture before it has a chance to evaporate. But in acne-prone skin a moisturizer like this will very often clog up the pores and provoke an outbreak of pimples. In my opinion, the solution is to use a urea-based moisturizer, whose chemical properties will attract and hold skin moisture without being sticky or occlusive.

Of course, attitudes toward bathing vary among cultures. In some societies it's customary to bath only once a week, or once a month. Most Americans bathe once a day, because whether or not stale perspiration odor offends the hearty French peasants of Burgundy (or whomever you care to cite as an example), it does happen to offend most of us. Like it or not, we are all products of a culture that puts a premium on cleanliness and attractive odors. The daily bath or shower is also a ritual that most of us don't want to give up, dry skin or no.

During summertime or in tropical climates, moisture in the air makes skin dryness less noticeable. But during the winter, when we're inside centrally heated homes and offices—where most of the moisture in the air has been fried away on hot radiators—skin can become flaky, itchy, peeling, or cursed with that very unattractive cracked mosaic look. This latter effect often shows up on women's legs, largely due to a combination of skin dryness and shaving. It's quite normal even among women whose skin is not particularly dry.

General advice for people with dry skin is to bathe with less frequency during the winter. Take your shower or bath every other day if you can, and make them shorter. It is always better to take a shower, which is less drying than total immersion in a tubful of water.

I don't want to give you advice that is incompatible with the widely held desire to feel clean and fresh-smelling every day. Instead, I want to teach you how to use your bath or shower to moisturize your skin. The hotter the water, for instance, the more the skin will be dehydrated. I know it feels grand to soak for hours in steaming water, but if your skin is dry, this will lead to considerable discomfort. Keep the water a little on the cool side of lukewarm. And *always* use bath oil.

Let me interject here that people who use bath oil slip and fall in the tub much more often than people who don't. But this is no excuse not to use bath oil; just be careful. Alpha Keri, Sardo, Johnson's Baby Oil, and almost any other bath oil will do the job excellently. If you're of a more economic turn of mind, you can make your own bath oil out of mineral oil (available at any druggist's), or even Wesson oil (or any other cooking oil) scented with as many drops of your favorite perfume as you deem desirable. A man with dry skin problems can scent mineral oil with his own cologne or aftershave and get the same results. A last word of advice: Use twice as much bath oil as the bottle tells you. I sometimes suspect that the various manufacturers want us to feel their products will go an extra-long way and so purposely tell us to use less than necessary.

The dry-skinned bather should not stay in a bath more than five minutes. If you don't have a clock in sight of the tub, then bring in a timer. And don't forget that the more water on your skin, the greater the drying action. Which is why showers, by definition involving less water, are preferable.

Now the following advice is for everyone, whether or not you have a dryness problem. It concerns the importance of using two types of soap. Palmolive Gold, Dial, or Irish Spring are great for odor problems, but they won't do anything for acne problems. Oilatum,

Tone, or Basis are very good for dry facial skin, but they aren't much help with malodorous armpits. My advice is to consider the needs of your face separately from those of the rest of the body. If logic indicates that you should wash with two different types of soap, then do so. This usually means washing your face in the sink either before or after your bath. If you have an acne problem but otherwise normal or slightly dry skin, then wash the face (or shoulders, thighs, or other acne-affected areas) with a drying acne soap like Fostex, Acnaveen, SAStid, Sulphur Soap, Acne-Aid, or Neutrogena. Then use Ivory, Palmolive, Caress, or whatever suits your pleasure for the rest of your body. If your face is dry and threatens to crease up with pseudo-wrinkles (temporary wrinkles due to tissue dehydration) while the rest of you is fighting an odor problem, then wash the face with Kauma, Alpha Keri, Tone, or Basis, and take a bar of Palmolive Gold into the tub with you. If you're showering, keep two appropriate bars of soap in the soap dish at all times. I like the products mentioned above, but they're chosen from a field of many others that are just as good. The point I'm trying to stress is that your face quite often needs a different soap from the rest of your body.

In the chapter on skin machines, I discussed the concept of epiabrasion, or vigorous scrubbing of the face. This is good for everybody, be their skin dry or oily, young or old. Use an appropriate soap and wash your face vigorously. This will not promote dryness if a good moisturizer is used after the bath. A final word of caution for bathers: Often a residue of soap remains on the skin and causes irritation of the underarms, waist, and groin area. If you favor the tub over the shower and suffer from this occasional irritation, then follow your bath with a thirty-second shower in cool-to-luke-warm water to rinse off any remaining soap.

The often divergent needs of the face and the body should concern everybody. But dry-skinned people should pay particular attention to the first five minutes after the bath. This is the crucial time in which to assure moisturization and to avoid dehydration. First, don't rub yourself dry. Instead, pat the excess water from face and body. Now, with the skin clean and freshly hydrated, apply a moisturizer all over. Almost any oil-based moisturizer is good for almost any body (not face). Nivea, Aquaphore, Eucerine, and Shepard's Lotion are a few of my favorites, but there are hundreds of others equally good. For that matter, you can rub in more of the bath oil you used in the tub for equally good moisturizing results.

Be sure, however, not to overdo it. Don't grease yourself down for a swim across the English Channel. Use just enough so that it vanishes into the skin. The effect of oil-based moisturizers is to seal moisture into the skin. This pore-clogging action is why young (and usually acne-prone) women especially must be careful of moisturizers on the face. As I said earlier, I'm a great believer in the chemical properties of urea, an aquaphilic substance that attracts and holds moisture without clogging pores. Aquacare, Carmol, and Neutraplus are examples of excellent urea-based moisturizing preparations that I particularly recommend for young or acne-troubled women.

Several Modified Bathing Methods

Here are six specific bathing regimens for more particular skin problems.

Zizmor's Modified Schultz Regimen: The Schultz Regimen was devised by a Dr. Schultz for people with excessively dry skin. It involves washing with a lipid-free (fat-free) lotion called Cetaphil, in lieu of soap and water bathing. Cetaphil is an excellent medication, requires no prescription, and simply will not cause skin dehydration. But a Schultz Regimen is a little extreme for all but the most serious dry skin problems. So, I suggest that you modify the regimen by alternating Cetaphil days with regular bathing days in whatever combination works best for you. For example, you might want to limit your regimen of short, cool showers and moisturizing to three days a week, and sponge yourself with Cetaphil on the other days. It depends on how dry your skin is. Fortunately, you can experiment with this lotion; it's very safe and is not going to hurt you.

Antifungal Baths: You can cure many fungal infections just by sitting in the bath. One of the most recalcitrant fungi is tinea versicolor. You may have it without even knowing it. At least, you won't know it until you take a sunbath, when it becomes dramatically obvious. Tinea versicolor fungi secrete a very effective sunscreen that prevents tanning. So even though it doesn't itch, it leaves you after a day of sunning with unattractive white blotches. Curiously, the fungus almost always spares the face. But the rest of you can look terrible.

A good home-remedy cure is to sit in a lukewarm to cool bath into which you have poured a cupful of vinegar. If the vinegar smell offends you, then add some of your favorite cologne. The vinegar's acidity will alter the pH of your skin, thereby disrupting the milieu in which the fungus thrives. Wash with a mild peeling soap—I like Stiefel Anti-Fungal Soap—to further rout out the fungus. You'll find that the Stiefel soap in the vinegar bath is also very effective against other fungal infections, especially in the groin area.

The Dead Sea Miracle Bath: You might have seen some of the recent publicity concerning psoriasis and eczema sufferers who experienced wonderful cures after bathing in the Dead Sea. The water there, like that of our own Great Salt Lake, is so salty that it actually feels oily to the touch. For reasons not fully understood, this super-salty water has helped not only psoriasis and eczema but also cracking dry skin problems.

You can duplicate the treatment by pouring a half box of coarse-grain kosher-type salt into your bath and soaking for five minutes. Pat yourself dry, combine with a sunlamp treatment (see Chapter 8 for details on sunlamps), and presto, you've re-created the Dead Sea!

Mud Baths: These are offered at fashionable spas, and the concept behind them is that minerals in the mud are somehow particularly nourishing to the skin. Mud baths are something like masks in that as they dry they promote a degree of beneficial peeling. This invigorates the skin and unclogs pores. Aside from that, I'm not so convinced that mud bath "minerals" or whatever can do much else.

But in the spirit of experimentation, I encourage you to try it yourself and see if you like it. And you needn't travel to an expensive Swiss spa when you can buy a bag of sterilized potting soil as near as the closest florist. Combine the soil with a half-milk–half-water solution until gummy. Put it on your face and body and let it dry for five minutes. Then wash it off in a quick cool shower.

The Sun Bath: A golden, long-lasting suntan, acquired without burning, just takes time. There are no short-cuts. If you're lucky, you might have inherited skin that tans easily, but that's in the hands of Mother Nature. And suntan preparation manufacturers can provide only limited help.

There is a relatively new chemical on the market, which has already been incorporated into the formulas of most suntan oils, creams, and lotions, called PABA (para-aminobenzoic acid). This is an astonishingly effective sunscreen that protects skin from burning even under intense tropical sun. It selectively screens out the sun's red rays, exactly those that cause burning and skin cancer.

On your first day in the sun, I would recommend that you apply a PABA sunscreen like Presun, Eclipse, or PabaGel to your entire body. Although this advice is intended for Caribbean vacationers more than suburban lawn-sitters, only you can assess the intensity of the sun and the sensitivity of your skin and decide what sort of protection you need.

Pure PABA will protect you from burning, but will also tend to retard tanning. On the other hand, regular suntan products containing PABA often don't contain enough to provide necessary protection on the first days of exposure.

My suggestion is to combine one of the PABA sunscreens with your favorite suntan product for a period of one week. On the first day, apply pure PABA. On successive days, use a mixture of gradually decreasing amounts of PABA with Coppertone or Bain de Soleil, or whatever you like. By the end of the week, you will have phased out the PABA entirely and be relying on the regular product.

People are always advised to severely limit the first few days of sun exposure. But with pure PABA on your skin, you drastically reduce the chances of a burn. Be sure to apply it to all sun-exposed areas, and not to forget the backs of your arms or the fronts of your legs or the tops of your feet. And if you go swimming, be sure to reapply the mixture to your entire body. One caution: PABA will stain white clothes yellow.

At the end of the day's sunning, moisturize the skin by taking a quick cool bath with lots of bath oil. Pat yourself dry and use a moisturizer (see page 45 for the appropriate moisturizer for your skin type.)

Zizmor's All-Purpose Compress: While on the subject of bathing, here is an excellent home remedy for almost any inflamed area. This is good for everything from poison ivy, to sunburn, to psoriasis, abrasions, minor cuts and scrapes, and so forth. It's better and cheaper than the first-aid creams in the drugstore.

Into a quart of cool water put two tablespoons of salt and a cup of skim milk (or two tablespoons of powdered milk). Shake it up, then soak a linen or any other suitable cloth in the mixture and wrap it over the affected area. The cloth need not be sterile. You'll find the effect very soothing.

10

Health and Beauty for Hands and Feet

Your hands take more abuse than any other part of your body. Between soap, sun, detergents, and home and industrial chemicals, it's not surprising that so many people have rough hands. Most hands have been doing nothing but hard work for most of our collective existence on the planet, except for members of that elite club called the aristocracy. For better or for worse, our historical fascination with (and sometimes ambivalence about) this soft-handed crew has left our culture with a longing for soft hands.

I want to put a few myths permanently to rest right now. The first myth is that washing is good for your hands. Wrong! Keeping your hands clean is good; washing them with unnecessary frequency is bad. For example, I commonly have patients who complain of ugly, itchy, scaly hand eczema. They are doubly perplexed, they say, because they wash their hands seven times a day! In fact, that's usually what's causing the eczema.

Of course you should wash your hands regularly, and if there's nothing wrong with them now, then there's little point in changing your hand-washing regime. But if you're suffering from dry, cracked, irritated, reddened, and uncomfortable hands, then the first thing you should do is wash them less.

Soap is strong, especially the tough stuff you find in institutional rest rooms. Dishwashing detergent is hard on hands too, so if you've been soaking in it, for heaven's sake stop! Too much washing can scrape away too many layers of cells, thereby removing vital barriers between you and your environment. If you have dry hands, but feel you must wash them more than twice daily, then use one of the superfatted soaps like Basis or Oilatum, which won't parch the hands.

Another widely accepted myth concerns the soothing properties of white liquid hand lotions. Although they smell divine and soothe like heaven for about five minutes, the sad truth about lotions is that they ultimately dry the skin. Hand lotions cannot provide lasting protection because they evaporate and destroy existing moisture, leaving the hand drier than it was in the first place.

If you're having a bout with wintertime dryness or dishwasher's hands, you'll find relief with either a cream or an ointment. I think everyone can recognize a cream, but the characteristic of an ointment is a greasy, jellylike consistency (Vaseline is a good example). Ointments provide more protection than creams because they are oilier and tend to stay on longer. I think Aquaphore is very good, as is plain old cooking Crisco. You can also ask your druggist for hydrophilic petrolatum, a compound that he keeps behind the counter and usually sells for a very reasonable price.

Some people find ointments too oily, so for them I would advise a cream. Creams have less staying power, but they usually don't feel greasy, nor are they expensive. I think the best hand cream around is Neutrogena Hand Cream, but it's a tie between that and Paquin. Also good and very popular is Nivea.

Zizmor's Special Dry Hand Regimen

Cutting down on washing and using a good cream or ointment still might not be enough to prevent dry hands. Women raising babies and cooking meals all day, secretaries (especially those working around Xerox machines), and men with jobs in certain chemical industries are all prone to dry hands and should use a miraculous little item called a fingercot.

A fingercot looks something like a miniature rubber condom, and you can buy them cheaply by the hundreds in a drugstore. They are of great value for cracked and excessively dry fingertips. Put a dab of cream or ointment on each fingertip, pull on the fingercots, and go about your business. You'll be able to type, use the telephone, cook, perform all your usual daily tasks quite comfortably. At the same time, the fingercots will be giving your parched fingertips a deep moisturization.

Even normally ineffective lotions work very well, since they can't evaporate inside a fingercot.

Rubber gloves are not very useful for dry hand care. Oftentimes they're clumsy, or else the rubber will cause an allergic irritation on sensitive hands. Besides, they're so occlusive that they can cause one of the sweat retention syndromes described in Chapter 5. A better idea for the care and prevention of rough hands is to adopt a nightly (or as often as practicable) ointment-and-bag ritual. Before you go to bed, rub your favorite cream or ointment into the hands, then put each hand into a plastic bag and tie with string at the wrist. If you can keep them on for an hour, fine; if you can keep them on all night, so much the better. The advantage of plastic bags is that some air can get inside, so they won't become too occlusive.

Some Thoughts on Washing Dishes

This is a practically insoluble problem. Dish-washing detergents are not only tougher than grease and dried-on food, they're tougher than your skin too! Rubber gloves help, assuming you can wear them and still hold on to the dishes. The best advice I can give is to rub an ointment well into the hands before you do the dishes, and repeat again when you're finished. Beware of hand lotions; used by themselves they'll only make dryness worse.

Age Spots and Sun Damage

Those brownish "liver spots" and reddish sun-damaged areas can be very disturbing. People feel that these marks make them look older, and they do. Although hands are very susceptible to sun damage, most of us go through life doing little to protect them. We usually even forget to put suntan lotion on the tops of our hands. And if there was ever anything that needed PABA protection, hands are it.

Fortunately, even if the damage has already been done, you can do lots to reverse or even eradicate it. Your first stop should be at your dermatologist's. Liver spots can be removed by a variety of techniques, including chemical burning, freezing, and simple scraping. They are not something you have to live with for the rest of your life.

As for sun-damaged areas, there is an excellent and fairly new topically applied prescription drug called Efudex. It contains 5-fluorouracil, an intriguing chemical that seeks out disorganized and cancerous skin tissue. It selectively destroys the errant cells while leaving surrounding tissue alone. The drug can even tell if certain areas that look fine now will show signs of sun damage in the near future. When damaged and disorganized cells are destroyed, fresh new skin will grow, and eventually an even skin tone will be restored.

Four Common Rashes

The first major category of hand rashes is related to excessive sweating. I refer you to Chapter 5 for a thorough discussion of what the rashes look like and what to do about them.

The next category of rashes occurs on the backs of the hands. When I see anything like this, I immediately think "photo-eruption," which means an eruption caused by a combination of the sun and something else. Diet sodas, certain soaps, water pills, some of the tetracyclines used in acne therapy, birth control pills, and various diabetic and high blood pressure medications are only a few of the things that, combined with sunlight, can cause rashes. If you're suffering from a rash like this, keep your hands out of the sun and make an appointment with your doctor. Possibly one of his prescriptions is causing the problem. And anyway, he'll be the most help in discovering which substance is the culprit.

But perhaps your problem is thickened reddened palms, accentuated hand markings, and generalized scaling and itching? If these symptoms are combined with similar symptoms on the feet, chances are you have a fungus infection. Steroid creams are often incorrectly prescribed for these problems. The creams do alleviate the itching somewhat, but they don't get to the source of the problem. The fungus doesn't go away, the symptoms persist, and finally the sufferer turns up at the dermatologist's office. If it is a fungus infection —which can be easily verified from a skin culture—it can be swiftly and completely eradicated by an OTC drug called Tinactin. If you recognize the above symptoms, then try Tinactin before you spend money on a visit to the doctor.

Finally, we have a rash called herpes simplex of the fingers. This herpes is a kissing cousin of the fever blister and venereal sore herpes, and like them it has painful symptoms and no cure. It is characterized by multiple-grouped little blisters that really hurt. As the episode advances, the whole arm begins to hurt and the armpit swells. Anybody can get it, but people who work on other people's mouths—dentists, dental hygienists, nurses—seem strangely susceptible. Sometimes sun exposure is thought to trigger the chain of reactions. As with the other herpes, nobody really understands the specific cause and effect relationships at work.

Although there is no cure for herpes simplex of the fingers, you can get some relief by application of the all-purpose compress described in Chapter 9 (p. 78). And don't be frightened by the enlarged lymph node in the armpit; it goes away.

The Skin on Your Feet

Naturally, this book makes no attempt to cover bone problems or aching feet. As far as the skin on the feet goes, almost every problem involves fungal infections, rashes, and eczema.

The most common fungal infection is athlete's foot, which is characterized by fissuring between the toes, especially between the fourth and fifth toes. The cure is simply to kill the fungus, which is easy to do by changing the ecology of the foot. Tinactin and Desenex are both good foot medicines. Follow the directions on the can, and keep the feet as dry as possible.

Sometimes you'll have a rash on the top of the foot without the characteristic fissuring between the toes that is associated with athlete's foot. In a surprising number of cases the rashes are caused by an allergy to the rubber construction in the toe of the shoe. We call this rubber box toe, and the prescription is to go out and buy a different pair of shoes.

Finally, there's eczema. I see this mostly on children, and it's often accompanied by similar rashes behind the knees or in the arm fold in front of the elbow. Your doctor will prescribe a steroid cream.

11

Buying Cosmetics and Using the Beauty Magazines

Buying cosmetics intelligently is a matter of knowing where to go and remembering that you get what you pay for. Let me reiterate that a good drugstore, although a vanishing species, is the best source of cosmetics. I offer the following suggestions for locating one. First, the cheapest is not necessarily the best. A drugstore with a large selection of competing brands, a pick-up and delivery service, medical prescription files on regular customers, and a well-trained and highly visible pharmacist on duty costs more to run. So, the prices are apt to be higher than at a discount drugstore.

However, I think a reliable drugstore is always worth

the extra cost. Remember, it's not just cosmetics you're buying here but prescription and over-the-counter medicines as well. Which is why you should choose a pharmacy with the same care you choose a doctor.

What are some things to beware of? Ironically, the big-volume cut-rate houses are only cheaper for the most common items, such as Valium, Librium, tetracycline, or Darvon. If you are buying more unusual drugs, you might actually spend more than you would at the corner chemist. Furthermore, many times you won't be able to find what you want if it's the least bit out of the ordinary.

One of my pet peeves is the know-nothing man in the white coat who questions everything your doctor told you. If you're dealing with a good pharmacist and he has a question about the medication, as a matter of course he'll telephone your doctor and get the answer from him. A good pharmacist will also explain to you how to use any prescription item you purchase. Beware the man who flamboyantly challenges the competence of your doctor; he might not know how to prepare your prescription.

I would advise you to steer clear, if possible, of drugstores that do a large Medicaid or union health plan business. These establishments operate on principles of high volume and little service. No union or government body is going to pay top-of-the-line prices for medication, so you can more or less count on getting second-best medications, if you can even find what you're looking for. Many a nurse or teacher who patronizes this type of establishment will give the pharmacist an extra dollar to do a careful job on a prescription. That's because the union that pays the bill doesn't.

A good drugstore with a highly qualified pharmacist will also have a wide selection of cosmetic lines. Sometimes, you'll have the option of a less expensive house brand too. The salespeople are often middle-aged or older ladies who are tremendously talented at exerting considerable sales pressure. That's a big reason for making cosmetic shopping a two-trip expedition: the first time without any money, the second time with no more than ten dollars. Let's face it, a great many cosmetic purchases are the result of impulse buying. The seductive packaging, the lure of a more beautiful you, the subtle pressure to buy, all make it hard to resist. So cultivate your resistance before you even approach the cosmetic counter.

A first-class drugstore will have plenty of mirrors, an atmosphere of comparative privacy, and a well-made-up salesperson who won't be overly coercive. Don't be afraid to touch, spray, or put on anything. Ask for advice on products produced by competing manufacturers (keeping in mind the medical advice contained in this book). The presence of competing brands is one of the best things about a good drugstore.

It's quite a different experience buying cosmetics from one of the big department stores. The trick there is not to get stuck at any one counter, where you will see the goods of only one manufacturer. Check everything out. Good stores usually have literally every cosmetic line. If you can't find exactly the shade you want, or a water-based formula for your acnegenic skin, or a nonocclusive moisturizer, then be sure and examine the competing counter across the aisle.

The drawbacks to department store buying are just the things to send you hurrying back to that wonderful sixty-years-on-the-same-corner drugstore. The atmosphere in department stores is not relaxed, no matter how elegant the store may be. Sometimes the prices are even a bit higher than elsewhere, especially if the store considers itself chic. And the custom-cosmetic counters, while offering a dazzling variety, will often sell you a product or particular color that you will never again be able to buy. In this case, as in so many others, highly fashionable means highly changeable.

On the plus side, department stores often give cosmetics away for free. "Buy $5 of this, and get another $5 worth of cosmetics for free," or at least a tote bag! Good stores will also schedule regular events at which guest makeup artists will teach you all sorts of clever tricks of the trade for free. Some of the big cosmetic houses present beauty courses right on the floor. These are generally inexpensive and can teach you how to make yourself over.

I recommend that you keep an eye on what's happening in the big store in town, but that you make your regular purchases at the same drugstore that supplies your medical needs. You'll get to know the people there, and if the products don't perform, you'll have somebody to complain to who'll actually listen. And if you see a lower price at a department store, your druggist will usually meet it if you are a good customer.

As for cheap cosmetics, I have nothing against them.

I believe in experimentation and the ability of the various government monitoring agencies to assure that nothing dangerous gets marketed in the dime store. Sometimes, it will be difficult to find exactly the right shade of, say, nail polish. But the cost is often substantially less. So by all means shop the dime stores and don't turn up your nose at the low prices.

Now I want to talk about the beauty magazines, of which I am very fond. Perhaps nowhere else is so much hope generated by the interaction of appearance and reality. These magazines churn out a tremendous amount of advice each month. But no matter how interesting and informative the articles, be sure to keep a few grains of salt by your reading light. The magazines are not the absolute last word on things. And they're not going to make you as beautiful as the models in their photographs. Many models aren't very attractive off camera anyway, and suffer from depressingly familiar things like bad skin. There's even a diet editor on one of the big magazines who weighs nearly two hundred pounds! Which only goes to say that you can't trust anybody all of the time.

However, if you don't let your ego become too battered by all that glamour, they're fun to read and full of useful information. I would suggest here that since beauty hints are found in other publications besides fashion magazines, you add health, sport, or nutrition publications to your monthly magazine shopping list. For example, *Prevention* magazine is filled with interesting articles on everything from nutrition to the latest studies on cancer. In between, you can usually find a number of ideas to help make you healthier and more attractive.

Vogue, Mademoiselle, Glamour, Seventeen, Harper's Bazaar carry excellent ideas on hairstyles, clothing, and diets. The diet departments are particularly inventive. They all help you to stay fashionable and conversant with the latest products from the big cosmetic houses.

12

Choosing and Using Dermatologists and Cosmetologists

How does a person become a dermatologist? He or she must first complete four years of undergraduate college, another four years of medical school, and three years of residency in dermatology at a hospital. After that comes a one-year apprenticeship of sorts, spent either in the hospital or in a private office. These are the minimum requirements. There's another logical step, however, that you should expect your dermatologist to have taken. This involves applying to the American Board of Dermatology for certification, a voluntary procedure described in Chapter 7.

A properly trained dermatologist can perform surgery,

administer injections, apply chemicals, prescribe treatment modalities that include X rays, freezing, sunlamps, and so on. Like so many other fields, dermatology has become highly specialized. And if you want a specialized treatment, search for a person with lots of experience doing the thing you want done. For instance, there's a doctor in my office building who does nothing but eye debagging. He's fully licensed to do other things, but he's so good at eyes that he's developed a large practice purely from word-of-mouth recommendations. There's another man on the West Coast who specializes in blistering skin diseases, a not-well-understood area that many doctors are reluctant to treat. There are people who do nothing but hair transplants, others who specialize in face peelings, and still others who have been doing new work with fibrin foam. My point, and I can't stress it enough, is that if you desire something specific, search for a dermatologist who's a specialist in that area.

Of course people come to dermatologists for more than cosmetic procedures. Bumps, warts, rashes, bad acne, and all manner of frightening and unfamiliar lesions can be treated by a dermatologist. It is customary to go to your regular family doctor first, who will then refer you to the dermatologist if need be. Not all, but certainly many of a dermatologist's patients are there because of a doctor's referral.

But not everybody has a doctor to refer them to a dermatologist. An alternative is to ask friends for a recommendation. Of course, all your friends may have perfect skin and no experience with a dermatologist. In this case, call your local county medical society and ask them to recommend a board-certified person with a conveniently located office. The assumption is that a good doctor will not only be board certified but will also be a member in good standing of his or her local county medical society.

There are other things besides office location and convenient hours to ascertain before you confirm an appointment. You have a right to ask the following questions, so don't be shy or intimidated. First, inquire about fees. What's the cost of a first consultation and how much are subsequent visits? If you're searching for a specific cosmetic procedure, does this doctor do a lot of it? You'll want to verify his board certification, and find out if he's associated with a good hospital. A hospital association means that the doctor spends at least a few hours a week working there, usually for free. This service is taken in many quarters not only as a demonstration of dedication to medicine for medicine's sake but also as another measure of the doctor's competency. In my opinion, you should stay away from a doctor with no hospital association. It may mean that he's too busy to spare the time or that no hospital wants his association; whatever it means, it rarely bodes well for you.

You can also inquire whether the dermatologist teaches anywhere. If he does, it's another good sign. It means not only that he has kept up with the latest developments in the field but also that he has met another set of exacting qualifications. Believe me, it's hard to get on the staff of a good teaching hospital. And it's a credit to the ability of any doctor who does.

You can do a bit more advance research on your

dermatologist by looking him or her up in the *Directory of Medical Specialists,* which can be found in any public library. This is a multivolume reference guide that's published every few years by Marquis, the people who bring out *Who's Who.* It indexes medical people three ways: alphabetically, by location, and by specialty. You can find out all about the dermatologist's professional history, outstanding publications, family, kids, and military service. You should expect any well-qualified practitioner to be listed there. The only exception might be young doctors who have made their reputations or started their practices in between editions.

I think it might be useful to give you a doctor's view of "a visit to the doctor." A dermatologist, like any medical person, is selling his time. You should expect adequate attention, but not an hour's worth of it. Somewhere between ten and thirty minutes is more than adequate for almost any first visit. If you've waited ten days for what turns out to be a ten-minute visit, don't feel slighted.

On the other hand, a doctor running an efficient office will not be excessively late when you're on time. Nor will he have a waiting room bursting with patients. The doctor can only see one person at a time, so it's pointless to pile patients up like that. Besides which, patients usually feel more comfortable and much less pressured in an uncrowded waiting room.

Openness and honesty must characterize your face-to-face meeting with the dermatologist. When he asks you to take off your clothes, even though you just have a wart on your finger, there's a good reason, so don't be embarrassed. Any skin doctor worth his or her salt will examine the *whole* skin, not just the problem that brought you to the office. It's amazing what else a doctor sometimes finds. Especially when there are lesions on the genitals, many patients are too modest to bring the subject up.

Don't think the doctor is prying when he asks you what medications you take (it's a good idea to bring the bottles with you), the state of your general health, your menstrual history, the names of your other doctors, and what previous treatments you've undergone. It is time to be worried if he *doesn't* ask you these questions. If he wants to know whether you've been to another dermatologist, tell the truth. If I see a patient with a bad acne problem, for example, it helps to know whether she's been to see Dr. so-and-so, who's widely known to prescribe such-and-such. The doctor's questions contribute to a fuller picture—what's wrong with you, and what's been done so far to correct it.

In too many cases a dermatologist will evaluate a given problem, give the patient a prescription, tell him or her to make another appointment in two weeks, and never see that patient again. Follow-up visits are important to evaluate progress, and sometimes to modify treatment. If you can't come back in two weeks, tell that to the doctor right away. I'll often prescribe completely different treatments for people I know I won't have an opportunity to see for a year than for those I know will be back in two weeks. If a patient tells me he or she cannot afford regular visits, I respect and appreciate their honesty. It makes it easier for both of us and insures the most efficient treatment modality.

Sometimes when a patient has an adverse reaction to prescribed medicine, instead of making another appointment, or at least calling the doctor's office, she or he will simply stop taking the medicine. This means the patient is out the money for the office visit and doesn't even get the benefit of the treatment. Always call your doctor if you have a problem with his therapy.

I want to urge every reader of this book to be a good patient. Don't change your appointment a dozen times. And changing a five o'clock appointment at five minutes to five is just as bad as not showing up at all. Doctors are people, too, and we appreciate patients who are on time and who pay their bills. I'm sure there are many of you who have been insulted when the doctor's receptionist insists that you pay for the visit before you walk out the door. This is a practice that is purely the result of the shockingly high proportion of patients who ignore doctor bills. It's too bad that so many honest bill payers have to get the C.O.D. treatment, but it's not meant personally. So if this is the practice at your dermatologist's office, I urge you not to be offended and to understand the reasons behind it.

While we're on the subject of money, your doctor will greatly appreciate your courtesy if you discuss your insurance before any work is done. If you ask him to accept assignment of the bill to Blue Cross, Blue Shield, Medicaid, Union Health, or whatever insurance you have, you're asking him to agree to accept whatever these com-

panies decide to pay. Sometimes an insurance policy will
specify a deductible amount that must be paid by you
before any benefit schedule goes into effect. In this case,
if you don't pay the deductible (and many people don't
know they have to), the doctor might not get paid at all.

Cosmetology and dermatology are services that
ideally complement one another. The big skin salons—
Georgette Klinger, Christine Valmy, Elizabeth Arden,
and so forth—are cosmetology houses. In addition to
national operations such as these, most cities of any size
will have individual practitioners who are sometimes
very talented.

Some states license cosmetologists and some don't.
The point of licensing is to attempt to assure the public
that the practitioner has some knowledge of skin and
is a person of good character. I agree with this concept;
given the choice, it's always preferable to deal with someone who is licensed.

Many of the treatments you'll receive at a skin salon
or at the office of an individual cosmetologist are excellent for acne problems. Cosmetologists often spend two
or three times as much time with you, for one-half to
one-third of the fee charged by a dermatologist. They
clean out pores, squeeze out blackheads and pimples,
deep-moisturize the skin with special steam mist machines, apply wonderful-feeling facial masks, and lavish
you with personal attention. Why is the cost so low? Because they usually exert considerable—albeit subtle—
pressure on you to buy cosmetics. And cosmeticians
make handsome profits on their cosmetics.

If I have a patient undergoing treatment for acne, I often recommend supplementary visits to a cosmetologist. These visits not only make the patient feel pampered but they reduce the number of times she needs to see me. Many dermatologists don't have time to clean out pores and blackheads, nor do they all offer advice on artistic application of makeup. Cosmetologists do both and can teach you all sorts of clever tricks.

Even if there's nothing wrong with your skin, you can go to a cosmetologist, receive lots of attention, get a deep cleansing, a lesson in makeup, and come out looking and feeling like a million dollars. The ideal time for one of these visits is the night before a big date or important party. And as long as you don't buy a load of expensive cosmetics, the cost is really low—even in the exclusive high-fashion houses.

In addition to thorough skin cleansings, makeup lessons, and luxurious surroundings, cosmetologists will often be able to make great (if temporary) improvements on aged skin. They have machines and techniques to deep-moisturize the face and plump up the skin cells. Many establishments will also give a massage and remove unwanted hair.

Cosmetologists and dermatologists do disagree on some subjects. For example, cosmetologists feel that dermatologists use chemical preparations that are too strong, and they often don't believe in antibiotics for acne therapy; dermatologists, on the other hand, believe that many cosmetics cause acne. Still, you can combine the services of both these professionals to your advantage.

Most cosmetologists depend on personal referrals for business. They also advertise in magazines and newspapers as well as in the Yellow Pages. Check a variety of categories; if there's nothing under "cosmetologists," then look under "skin treatments," or something similar.

Because of their dependence on referrals, you'll usually find the cosmetology staff very solicitous and helpful. They want you to come back, preferably with your friends. They also want you to buy lots of cosmetics, but this is the last time I'll warn you on that score.

A final word: As I've mentioned before, in addition to big salons, there are many individual cosmetologists who practice out of small private offices. Sometimes these ladies—often older and of genteel European extraction —are absolutely great. They're just as helpful as the fashionable clinics and salons, so don't disregard them just because they haven't been featured in *Vogue*.

13

The Do-It-Yourself Skin Test

The following skin test is unique because it not only provides answers but also explains the purpose behind each question. You may have seen similar skin tests in salons or magazines, but now you'll discover why the doctor or cosmetologist was asking those questions. When you finish this test, you won't have to take out a mortgage to finance a sackful of expensive potions and cosmetics. Instead, you will have compiled a list of cross-references to chapters in this book that contain helpful do-it-yourself information tailored specifically to your type of skin.

Several admonitions are in order. First, don't go looking for trouble. It may well be that there is either nothing or not much wrong with your skin. In which case, be thankful. Second, no one else is evaluating this test but you, so don't be afraid to admit to unfashionable answers. Third, you may not fit clearly into any of the categories of answers that follow each question. This test is designed to be a tool to help identify and improve normal skin problems; it's not a substitute for medical care.

The test is divided into two sections. The first contains general questions whose aim is to provide a profile of your skin type and environmental surroundings. The second section should be performed naked in front of a mirror, and its goal is to help you visually locate cosmetic problem areas. So get your pencil ready and let's begin.

The Do-It-Yourself Skin Test

SECTION ONE: QUESTIONS

(Please complete the test before referring to the answers that follow it.)

1. How old are you?

2. What color is your skin?

3. What color are your eyes?

4. What color is your hair?

5. What skin and scalp conditions affect your immediate family?

6. Would you describe your skin as normal, oily, dry, or a combination of these?

7. Do you tan easily or get sunburned?

8. Are you taking any medicines?

9. Do you take birth control pills?

10. Are you nervous or under constant stress?

11. How much makeup do you use?

12. Approximately how many hairs do you lose each day?

13. How often do you bathe?

14. Does your home or office have sealed windows?

15. What is your height and weight?

16. How much sun do you get?

17. What is your occupation?

18. Is your menstrual cycle regular?

19. Do you have diabetes or a thyroid condition?

20. Do you eat fast foods?

21. Do you use artificial sweeteners?

22. Do you take vitamins?

23. Do you smoke?

SECTION ONE: ANSWERS

1. *How old are you?*

The commonest skin problem for persons twenty years old or younger is oiliness and acne. Acne in this age group responds exceedingly well to drying medicines that are applied to the skin surface. See Chapter 20, "Acne" and be comforted with the knowledge that teenage acne is the easiest to cure. Also helpful are the regimens contained in Chapter 14, "Oily Skin Regimens."

Persons between the ages of twenty and thirty-five often have two problems: oiliness and acne; and the beginning of dryness. Both these problems will often coexist on separate sections of the same face. The dry condition rules out the use of very tough acne medicines. Refer to the sunbath section of Chapter 9, "How to Take a Bath," Chapter 14, "Oily Skin Regimens," Chapter 15, "Dry Skin Regimens," and Chapter 20, "Acne."

Between the ages of thirty-five and fifty, oiliness usually declines, while dry skin and large pores become increasingly worrisome. The older you are, the more cautious you must be when sunbathing, so refer to the sunbath section in Chapter 9, "How to Take a Bath." Also see Chapter 15, "Dry Skin Regimens," and Chapter 17, "Large Pore Regimens."

Persons fifty and older usually have dry skin along with various combinations of wrinkles, spots, and old-age lesions. There's lots you can do to make things better, as can be seen in Chapter 7, "Cosmetic Surgery," Chapter 15, "Dry Skin Regimens," and Chapter 16, "Aging Skin: What to Do About It."

2. *What color is your skin?*

Fair and very fair skin often overreacts to drying acne medicines. This type is generally more prone to eczema, dryness, wrinkling, sunburn, skin cancer, or any kind of sun damage. Take to heart the sunbathing suggestions in Chapter 9, "How to Take a Bath," as well as the regimens in Chapter 15, "Dry Skin Regimens."

Most people, naturally, have a medium skin complexion. If there's nothing wrong with it, leave well enough alone.

Mediterranean complexions have a tendency to greater oiliness and related acne as well as enlarged pores. On the other hand, these persons have a much higher tolerance to sun exposure. See Chapter 17, "Large Pore Regimens," and Chapter 20, "Acne."

Black skin also generally tends to oiliness and enlarged pores. In addition, it suffers from keloidal scarring, blotchy darkening from certain acne medications, and a tendency to blotch after a skin inflammation. These problems are specifically dealt with in Chapter 21, "Black and Beautiful," as well as in Chapter 17, "Large Pore Regimens," and Chapter 20, "Acne."

3. What color are your eyes?

Blue, gray, green, and light brown eyes are usually the hallmark of fair-skinned people. So, beware the aforementioned dangers of sunburn, dryness, wrinkling, and skin cancer. See the sunbath section in Chapter 9, "How to Take a Bath," and Chapter 15, "Dry Skin Regimens," and perhaps Chapter 16, "Aging Skin: What to Do About It."

The darker shades of brown eyes usually complement dark complexions. Dark-complected people are not only more sun-tolerant but are also more susceptible to oiliness and acne. Helpful chapters include Chapter 9, "How to Take a Bath," Chapter 20, "Acne," and Chapter 21, "Black and Beautiful."

4. *What color is your hair?*

Your hair color also helps to classify you as either fair and dry or dark and oily. Blond, red, and light brown hair are usually associated with fair skin; brown and black usually go with darker complexions. See the appropriate chapters referred to in Question No. 3.

5. *What skin and scalp conditions affect your immediate family?*

A tendency toward acne, baldness, and allergies is largely a matter of the genes you carry. If either side of your family suffers from these conditions, then chances are you have a genetic makeup that makes you similarly susceptible. You can get a clearer idea of what's in store, or what you're already enduring, by referring to those of the following chapters that apply to you: Chapter 15, "Dry Skin Regimens," Chapter 18, "Heads Up! The Best Things to Do for Your Hair," Chapter 20, "Acne," and Chapter 23, "Seasonal Skin Care Reminders."

6. *Would you describe your skin as normal, oily, dry, or a combination of these?*

Oily skin is shiny, greasy, and probably suffers from at least some acne. Dry skin tends to itch, flake, sometimes scale, and almost always gets worse in the winter. Luckily, many people have normal, problem-free skin. If you're oily, dry, or have a combination of oily and dry patches, consult Chapter 14, "Oily Skin Regimens," and Chapter 15, "Dry Skin Regimens."

7. Do you tan easily, or get sunburned?

If you burn easily, chances are you've got fair skin. In addition to sunburn, you're probably a candidate for dryness and premature wrinkling. See Chapter 9, "How to Take a Bath," Chapter 15, "Dry Skin Regimens," and Chapter 16, "Aging Skin: What to Do About It."

If you tan well, you're fortunate and can proceed directly to the next question.

8. Are you taking any medicines?

Every pill you take—be it a vitamin, aspirin, or birth control pill—is a medicine. Certain medications can make acne worse (see Chapter 20, "Acne"), make hair fall out (see Chapter 18, "Heads Up! The Best Things to Do for Your Hair"), or cause photosensitizing reactions (see Chapter 2, "*The* Diet for Your Skin," and Chapter 9, "How to Take a Bath").

9. Do you take birth control pills?

A common exchange in my office goes as follows: Q. "Are you taking any medicines?" A. "No." Q. "Are you taking birth control pills?" A. "Yes." Repeat: Birth control pills are medicine. They can also make hair fall out, make acne worse (or better), and photosensitize the skin. I refer you to the chapters mentioned under Question No. 8, as well as Chapter 4, "Sex and Your Skin."

10. *Are you nervous or under constant stress?*

Nervousness, especially when it's protracted, can lead to a hormonal imbalance that causes an increase in oil secretion, which in turn can cause acne. Nervousness can also make you itch like crazy and cause your hair to fall out. If you're nervous and oily, see Chapter 14, "Oily Skin Regimens," and Chapter 20, "Acne." If you're nervous and itchy, see Chapter 15, "Dry Skin Regimens," and perhaps Chapter 4, "Sex and Your Skin." In any case, make it a point to calm yourself down.

11. *How much makeup do you use?*

While makeup can protect the skin over a lifetime, it can also cause acne. See Chapter 6, "The Art of Using Makeup," Chapter 17, "Large Pore Regimens," and Chapter 20, "Acne."

12. *Approximately how many hairs do you lose each day?*

A good way to find out is to count them after combing. One hundred to two hundred hairs per day is the normal rate of loss. If you exceed that, consult Chapter 18, "Heads Up! The Best Things to Do for Your Hair."

13. How often do you bathe?

Questions like this help determine if you're making an existing dry skin problem worse. Too much bathing dehydrates the skin. For the right and wrong ways to bathe, see Chapter 9, "How to Take a Bath," and Chapter 15, "Dry Skin Regimens."

14. Does your home or office have sealed windows?

This question also is aimed at unearthing contributing factors to a dry skin problem. A too-dry environment can turn a slight tendency to dryness into tormenting itchiness or worse. You should humidify your environment to help dry skin; see also Chapter 15, "Dry Skin Regimens."

15. What is your height and weight?

Be honest now! The following chart is included to help you ascertain whether or not you're overweight.

HEIGHT	DESIRABLE WEIGHT FOR WOMEN
5′ –5′2″	95–110 lbs.
5′2″ –5′4″	105–120 lbs.
5′4″ –5′6″	110–130 lbs.
5′6″ –5′8″	120–140 lbs.
5′8″ –5′10″	125–145 lbs.
5′10″–6′	140–160 lbs.

Fat people tend to perspire more, which can lead to a variety of skin complications. See Chapter 2, "*The* Diet for Your Skin," Chapter 3, "Fat Treatments and Cellulite," and Chapter 5, "Doctor, I Sweat All the Time!" Crash diets can wreak havoc with the complexion, so please heed the advice in Chapter 2, "*The* Diet for Your Skin."

16. How much sun do you get?

Too much sun can be unduly drying, particularly if you're older or fair skinned. Refer to Chapter 15, "Dry Skin Regimens," and Chapter 16, "Aging Skin: What to Do About It."

Too little sun only hurts if you suffer from dandruff, psoriasis, or eczema. If you do, see the suggestions in Chapter 18, "Heads Up! The Best Things to Do for Your Hair," and Chapter 20, "Acne."

17. What is your occupation?

This question is, again, designed to assess sun exposure and the humidity of your environment. For example, if you work indoors, you may be drying yourself out; if you're a tennis pro, you may be overexposing yourself to the sun. The question is primarily aimed at dry skin sufferers, so if that's you, see Chapter 15, "Dry Skin Regimens," for helpful suggestions.

18. *Is your menstrual cycle regular?*

Irregular menstrual patterns can mean hormonal problems, which can cause acne, hair loss, and so forth. See your doctor or dermatologist. Also, refer to Chapter 4, "Sex and Your Skin," Chapter 14, "Oily Skin Regimens," Chapter 18, "Heads Up! The Best Things to Do for Your Hair," and Chapter 20, "Acne."

19. *Do you have diabetes or a thyroid condition?*

Diseases *and* the drugs that are used to treat them can be responsible for hair loss, bad nails, photosensitization (in the case of diabetic medicines), dry skin, and anemia (in the case of thyroid problems). If these symptoms affect you, discuss your medication with your doctor.

20. *Do you eat fast foods?*

Well, there's nothing good about an unbalanced diet, but on the other hand, there's nothing wrong *per se* with fast foods. As far as your skin is concerned, about the only pitfall to fast foods is their high iodine content, which stems from the purveyor's commendable desire to maintain high standards of hygiene. Deep fryers are often sanitized with high-iodine solutions, and the iodine (not surpisingly) manages to get into the food. Iodine is linked to pustular eruptions in the skin, also known as acne. See Chapter 2, *"The* Diet for Your Skin."

21. *Do you use artificial sweeteners?*

The sweeteners in diet foods and sodas can photo-sensitize the skin. This means that they can induce a bad sunburn even on skin that's normally quite tolerant to sun exposure. This question, then, is designed to uncover a possible reason for sunburning. See the sun-bath section in Chapter 9, "How to Take a Bath."

22. *Do you take vitamins?*

Many multivitamin formulas are high in acnegenic iodine. See Chapter 2, "*The* Diet for Your Skin," and Chapter 20, "Acne."

23. *Do you smoke?*

For reasons not fully understood, smokers have a tend-ency to develop crows' feet around the eyes. See Chap-ter 7, "Cosmetic Surgery," and Chapter 16, "Aging Skin: What to Do About It."

SECTION TWO

Now comes the moment of truth. Take off your clothes and stand before a mirror. You should do this in the morning, before you bathe or apply makeup. The checklist that follows will help you pinpoint exactly where your skin needs help.

1. *Are you overweight?*

If so, this is as good a time as any to decide to do something about it. Refer to Question No. 15 in the previous section for the scale of height and desirable weight; and to Chapter 2, "*The* Diet for Your Skin," for sensible weight-loss programs.

2. *Is your face oily, dry, or both?*

I think Max Factor Blue Mask is an excellent way to discover exactly which areas of the face are overly oily and which are overly dry. It's also pleasant and easy to use. Or, you can tear a brown paper supermarket bag into handy scraps and rub them on the various portions of your face. Normal skin will leave an oily residue on brown paper. But if the paper becomes translucent, the area is too oily. If there is nothing at all on the paper, the skin area is probably too dry. The purpose of all this is to note exactly where the dry and oily areas are located on your face. Chapter 14, "Oily Skin Regimens," and Chapter 15, "Dry Skin Regimens," contain useful suggestions for each area.

3. *Is your face wrinkled?*

If so, see Chapter 16, "Aging Skin: What to Do for It."

4. Do you have acne?

There's lots to be done for pimples, blackheads, pustules, and so forth. See Chapter 20, "Acne."

5. Do you have large pores?

If so, refer to Chapter 17, "Large Pore Regimens."

6. Can you note brown aging spots?

Lesions associated with aging can appear on the face, hands, neck, torso, or any other part of the body. If you have aging lesions, you must be particularly cautious in the sun. See the sunbath section in Chapter 9, "How to Take a Bath." Suggestions on how to rid yourself of aging lesions can be found in Chapter 7, "Cosmetic Surgery," and Chapter 16, "Aging Skin: What to Do About It."

7. Are there visible veins on your skin?

Sometimes the cause is age, sometimes birth control pills, sometimes sun exposure, sometimes a combination of them all. See Chapter 4, "Sex and Your Skin," Chapter 7, "Cosmetic Surgery," and Chapter 16, "Aging Skin: What to Do About It."

8. Is the center of your face noticeably redder than the rest of you?

If so, you may be photosensitizing yourself with either birth control pills or artificial sweeteners. Consult your doctor.

9. Are there white blotches on your skin that won't tan?

You might be host to a fungus called tinea versicolor, harmless except for the fact that it secretes an extremely effective sunscreen. Washing with Stiefel Anti-Fungal Soap will get rid of it.

14

Oily Skin Regimens

Oily skin is a problem only if it's excessively oily. If your face is neither unattractively greasy nor besieged with continual acne flare-ups, then let well enough alone. Often the use of water-based cosmetics, rather than oil-based preparations, is the only precaution necessary. Water-based formulas in products by Mary Quant, Liqui-mat, and Clinique (to name only a few) will reduce the chances of clogging your pores. Chapter 20 describes in detail the direct relationship between clogged pores and acne pimples.

If, however, your skin is unpleasantly oily, you can substantially improve your situation with the regimens that follow. These regimens are graduated in intensity, and can be used individually or in combination with one another. You're the judge as to what works best on your own skin. Oiliness is a highly variable condition that affects different people in different degrees. Sometimes the entire face is oily; sometimes only portions are. It's up to you to experiment with the regimens in order to get the best results.

Now, a word on what causes oiliness in the first place. If you think it comes from eating too much pizza, deep-fried chicken, or french fried potatoes, you're mistaken. The oil and grease in your diet have no effect on oil secretion. The amount of sebaceous oil secreted onto the surface of your face is determined by genetics and hormones. If you come from an oily-skinned family, your inherited genes are the probable cause of your oiliness. To a great extent, your personal hormonal recipe is genetically determined. The male sex hormone androgen (found in men and women), as well as androgenlike hormones, and androgenic substances all stimulate oil secretion.

But it's quite easy to increase your level of secretion by eating androgenic foods (like wheat germ), taking certain kinds of birth control pills, and otherwise increasing the amount of androgen in your system. Eating oily foods, however, will not stimulate oil production.

Other things influence oiliness. Stress, for example, can trigger the adrenals in such a way as to hormonally induce excess oil production. Too much dryness can, ironically, do the same. Sometimes after chemical peeling, dermabrasion, or heavy doses of dehydrating sun exposure, the body's natural reaction will be to replace lost moisture with an abundant and perplexing (to the layman) rate of oil secretion. Cosmetics and hair preparations can also add a bit too much extra oil to an already moderately oily skin. The result can be pimples, greasiness, or pomade acne, which is the name for hair-line acne breakouts caused by pores clogged with hair preparations.

But, fortunately, oiliness can be controlled with easy physical and chemical modalities. As you proceed with the regimens that follow, be sensible and move cautiously. If you're fair, remember that fair-skinned, light-haired people normally react more strongly to sunlight and chemicals. And don't forget to start with milder regimens first, then work up to the more rigorous ones.

Regimen No. 1: The Twice-Daily Astringent

At the time when you might otherwise have a mid-morning snack or afternoon tea—10 A.M. and 4 P.M.—you can instead wipe problem oily areas with cotton balls soaked in an astringent. Ordinary isopropyl alcohol from any druggist is just fine, as is witch hazel. If you want something a little more elegant, try Seba-Nil towelettes, which are convenient and have a little scent. Also pleasant and effective are the various clarifying lotions sold by the major cosmetic houses. Another suggestion, particularly good if you've got a long-standing acne condition, is a medicated astringent. Your doctor can give you a prescription for 2 percent salicylic acid tincture. Salicylic acid is a peeling agent; the other 98 percent is alcohol.

Cleanse the oily areas of your face twice daily with whatever astringent most pleases you. Your skin should become clearer, and acne incidence should drop off considerably. Be sure to give the skin an opportunity to adjust to the new regimen. Initially, you may seem to become oilier, but this should be only temporary. If your skin becomes irritated, stop for a day or two to give the skin a chance to adapt. And please don't clog up your pores with heavy oil-based makeup after the astringent cleaning.

Regimen No. 2: The Soap and Water Ritual

I don't call this a "ritual" for nothing. I mean for you to do it religiously three times daily: on awakening, at lunchtime, and at bedtime. Run lukewarm to coolish water in the basin, wash the face with soap (see below) and a cloth, leave the lather on the face for a minute, and rinse. Then wash a second time but don't make the second rinse quite so thorough. You want to leave a very slight soap residue on the skin.

Your choice of soap must again be the result of experimentation. You'll want a drying soap, which you might like to choose from the following list.

Acnaveen	Neutrogena
Acne-Aid	Neutrogena Acne Soap
Fostex	SAStid
Ivory	Sulphur Soap
Lifebuoy	

Sometimes, it's a good idea to use the drying soap during only one of each day's three washings. You can use your favorite bath soap the other two times. Or, use the drying soap on two of the three washings. It depends on how much drying you want and on your own levels of skin tolerance.

Remember to let your face acclimate itself to this sort of vigorous degreasing. If it gets irritated, skip a day or two.

Regimen No. 3: Drying Shampoos

Your hair may be more oily than you realize. Many oily foreheads plagued with acne can be cleared up quite simply by a change of shampoo. The following all contain drying chemicals of one sort or another. They're available without prescription, so you can experiment to find the one you like the best.

Head & Shoulders   Vanseb-T
Sebulex   Zetar
Sebutone   Zincon
Selsun

This is a partial list; other products are available that will do the job just as well. Changing shampoos causes perhaps the least disruption in your normal beauty regimen. So if your oily skin problem exhibits symptoms of pomade acne, this will provide the simplest cure.

Regimen No. 4: The Once-a-Day Sunlamp Treatment

Basically, sun and sunlamp treatments have a twofold effect on the skin: They encourage a mild peeling that strips away oil plugs and unclogs pores; and they toughen the skin, thereby discouraging oil secretion.

Any brand of sunlamp will do. The only necessary accoutrements are opaque goggles or plastic cups to protect the eyes and a tube of zinc oxide paste (available at a drugstore) to protect the lips. It's important not to miss a day on a sunlamp regimen, so choose a convenient time that you can be relatively certain of having free every day.

The first day's exposure shouldn't last longer than five seconds. Move the face slowly from side to side and up and down to assure even exposure. Each day, increase the exposure time by five seconds. If you feel you're beginning to burn, then either skip the day's normal increment, or decrease the dosage by five seconds. You should stop the increments when you reach a plateau of between three and four minutes. At this point, not only should the oily problem be significantly reduced, but you'll also have a nice deep color.

It's most important not to skip even a single day. Sunlamp exposure causes a natural thickening of the skin; conversely, a lack of exposure will lead to a thinning. This alternation sometimes leads to acne outbreaks, so be assiduous and don't miss a day.

A balanced sunlamp regimen shouldn't cause any worries about burns or skin cancer. Sunlamps, when properly used, just aren't strong enough to cause cancer. In fact, many psoriasis patients regularly undergo sunlamp exposure that makes our regimen here look pale indeed. It doesn't hurt them, so your three-to-four-minute daily ritual won't hurt you either. At worse, you may experience a little pseudo-wrinkling caused by temporary skin dehydration. To clear this up, at the end of each treatment, pat the face with water and apply a urea-based moisturizer like Aquacare or Carmol.

Regimen No. 5: Get a Suntan

If the circumstances of your life are such that you can bask in the sun almost every day, then you have a ready-made course of action to counter oiliness. Since the sun's rays have a much longer-lasting effect than those of a sunlamp, you can more easily miss a day here and there without breaking out. Instead of five-second increments, adjust your time of exposure to the dictates of your local climate and life-style.

Now it is true that a lifetime's accrual of sun exposure can cause skin cancer. But it is also true that the new sunscreens that contain PABA (para-aminobenzoic acid) will screen out cancer-causing rays. Personally, I like Presun, PabaGel, and Eclipse, all very good PABA products in nonacnegenic alcohol bases. By applying these preparations before exposure, you can sit in the sun every day, enjoying not only a golden tan, but also a major decrease in skin-surface oil secretion, while you are protected from burning and cancer-causing sun rays.

Regimen No. 6: Cryo-exfoliation

This is the most rigorous of our oily regimens. You'll need a blender and some precipitated sulphur, an inexpensive nonprescription item available at any well-stocked drugstore. The idea here is to spot-freeze the skin's surface, causing a mini-peeling that will strip away oil plugs and open up pores.

Although a doctor uses dry ice in his office, you can use ice from your refrigerator. Crush it in the blender (or pound it in a cloth) until mushy, then wrap in cheese-cloth. Take a teaspoon of the sulphur, sprinkle evenly on a flat surface (a length of aluminum foil is good), and dab the cheesecloth ice pack onto the foil so as to get a nearly even coating of sulphur on a small section of the moist cloth. Press the sulphur-coated ice pack onto an oily area of the face until it feels mildly uncomfortable. Don't overdo it. When you remove the ice pack from your face, dab it again in the sulphur and press against the next oily area. Continue until all oil-troubled areas have been treated. Then wait five minutes, allowing the face to dry with the sulphur on it. The last step is to wipe the face clean with a washcloth soaked in isopropyl alcohol or any convenient astringent.

On account of the exfoliation (peeling) caused by the ice, and the drying action of the sulphur, this is considered a strong treatment. I doubt anyone could do it every day, so experiment and do it only when you feel the need.

15

Dry Skin Regimens

The medcial term for dry skin is "xerosis"—just, incidentally, as "Xerox" refers to a dry-copying process. Skin that's too dry tends to be red, rough to the touch, flaky, and itchy. People with dry skin usually feel better in the summer, for winter brings central heating that dehumidifies the interiors of many homes and offices. However, even during humid summer weather dry skin is still uncomfortable.

Skin on any part of the body can be dry. The manifestations of dryness go all the way from a little bit of redness and occasional scaling to a condition called atopic eczema. The Greek root of the word *atopic* means strange, which aptly describes the condition itself. People with skin this dry suffer from hardened tissue with accentuated skin markings, particularly in the creases behind the elbows and knees. The skin is thickened, maddeningly itchy, and can make you generally miserable.

Fortunately, not many people get severe cases. For most women, the worst symptom of dryness is an occasional crazed mosaic pattern on the legs, or a bit of itchy redness around the mouth.

But since many women have both dry and oily areas on the skin, choosing a treatment is confusing. What's called the "butterfly"—think of your nose as the body of a butterfly whose wings are spread out on both your cheeks—is usually oily, even on dry-skinned people. In contrast, the peri-oral area—the skin surrounding your mouth—is usually dry even on oily people. Some people do have dry butterflies and oily peri-oral areas, but they're in the minority.

People with dry faces should avoid drying agents such as cosmetic clarifying lotions, toners, and astringents. Drying chemicals contained in deodorant soaps and certain shampoos are to be avoided too. If dry skin is an all-over problem, shampoo in the sink, not in the shower where drying suds will get all over you. Since sun exposure is dehydrating, it also should be approached with care. However, it is a curious fact that sun exposure (short of sunburn) can actually help some dry-skin sufferers. The dehydration may stimulate additional oil secretion, but no one knows for sure.

Since excessive dryness and oiliness coexist on so many faces, I offer the following general advice. Younger or more acne-prone people should concentrate on their oily problem (see the regimens in Chapter 14), and treat dry areas with a urea-based nonocclusive moisturizer like Aquacare, Aquacare/HP, or Carmol. Conversely, older or less acne-prone people are advised to concentrate on the dry problem, for which I have designed the regimens in this chapter.

Before you judge yourself as dry, oily, or both, you'll want to determine extent, location, and seriousness of the condition. A good procedure you can do at home is the Brown Paper Test. All you need is a brown paper supermarket bag. The test should be conducted about half an hour after you get up in the morning (naturally before washing), when your skin is in its most natural state. Tear off small pieces of paper and smear them over various portions of your face. You'll be able to see the oil darken the paper, which is quite normal. But if the paper actually becomes translucent, then that area is too oily.

Perhaps a better idea is to buy a tube of Max Factor Blue Mask. This relatively new product is pleasant to use, and when the mask is peeled off, you can easily see which parts of the face are too dry and which are too oily. Flakes of skin will adhere to the mask where it touches excessively dry areas, whereas the too-oily areas make the mask a darker blue. It's a good product that does its job well.

Two final suggestions: Go to a dermatologist or avail yourself of the free skin analyses offered at many of the cosmetology salons. The dermatologist can give you the most professional opinion plus any necessary medical prescriptions. A salon visit involves a trained cosmetologist who examines your face and draws you a little chart showing where the oily and dry areas are located on your face. But while the skin analysis is often free, you're expected to purchase cosmetics. You don't have to, but it is expected.

I do want to stress that if your skin is not bothering you, you don't need a dry skin regimen. Having said that, I will now give you a few examples of dry skin problems that most people think are caused by something else. The first is redness and irritation around the eyes and eyelids. This is almost never caused by eye makeup, which is tested with great thoroughness precisely so that it won't be irritating. Usually these symptoms are due to dry skin in the eye area, which is easily treated with almost any moisturizer. Similarly, many a patient with a red and itchy neck is convinced that she has an allergy to her silver necklace or wool sweater. But again it's usually just a matter of dry skin. Sometimes older people enter a hospital with perfectly fine skin, then get redder and itchier by the day. All too often they think they're allergic to their medication, when actually it's just the arid hospital environment that's drying out their skin. Even experienced doctors can misinterpret these symptoms.

"Why me?" you may ask. In most cases, dry skin is a matter of heredity. In many other cases, you may be causing the condition yourself by overwashing your face or overtreating an acne problem with extremely drying acne medicines. Although sun exposure does help some dry-skinned people, its usual effect is to dehydrate the skin, making dryness worse. If you swim in chlorinated pools, take too many saunas, or live in the desert, your skin may become dry. Similarly, water pills or one of the several types of birth control pills can also lead to drying of the skin. Nicotinic acid, prescribed for blood vessel diseases, is one of the numerous obscure drugs that are drying. If the onset of dryness seems to coincide with any new course of medication that you're on, ask your doctor if there's a correlation.

The key to regulating dry skin is controlling your environment. Here are three regimens to help you do exactly that. Use them either individually or together, as needed. Experiment, and don't give up before your skin has a chance to improve.

Regimen No. 1: Humidifying the Environment

You don't have to move to the tropics to live in a less dry environment. Even if there's nothing you can do about an office environment, there's lots you can do to humidify your home. The first step is to buy a small electric humidifier and put it in the bedroom (or wherever you spend the most number of hours). If the bathroom is near your bedroom, keep the tub filled with a few inches of water when it isn't being used. Throughout your house or apartment, set out shallow tubs or trays of water and make it an evening ritual to fill them. All these water surfaces will gradually evaporate into the air, making it more moist and beneficial to your dry skin.

There's more you can do. Since coolness is good for dry skin, never set your thermostat above 67 degrees. If you live in an overheated apartment where you can't control the steam, then keep the windows open a crack when the heat is on. Another good idea is to buy plants and keep them well watered and misted. Greenery helps to moisten the environment through transpiration, the emission of water from the leaves of plants. (P.S.: I'm told that overwatering is the major cause of death among house plants, so be careful!)

Regimen No. 2: The Cool Bath

The ideal temperature for this bath should be 76 degrees (never above 84 degrees). I have discussed bathing in greater detail in Chapter 9. For now I just want to remind dry-skinned bathers to keep the number of weekly baths they take to an absolute minimum. Water immersion and subsequent drying dehydrates the skin, exactly what you can't afford. If possible, take a shower. But whichever you take, make it short and cool. Take a thermometer and test your bath water; learn what 76 degrees feels like. If you can stand the temperature a bit lower, so much the better.

Always use bath oil, which you'll be glad to know makes cool water feel warmer. Alpha Keri, Kauma, and Jeri Bath Oil are all good, as are any number of others. Don't use a drying soap (never a deodorant bar), but stick instead to Oilatum, Basis, Dove, Tone, Caress, or anything else that contains bath oil or cream. You won't feel squeaky clean when you get out of this bath, but remember that squeakiness results when natural oils have been stripped away. Pat yourself dry, and immediately apply a moisturizer. Younger or acne-prone women should use a nonocclusive moisturizer containing urea. These preparations will attract and hold moisture without clogging and sealing pores like the oil-based moisturizers. My favorite urea-based moisturizers are Aquacare, Aquacare/HP (which contains more urea), and Carmol (with yet more urea).

Regimen No. 3: Moisturizing the Face

This is a once-a-day morning ritual to be done just after you wake up. Run very hot tap water onto your washcloth, wring it out, spread it over the face, and leave on for about a minute so that the heat can open up your pores. Then pat the face dry, leaving a few beads of water, and apply a moisturizer. Younger women should stick to the aforementioned urea products; if you're older and haven't had a pimple in twelve years, then you can use an oil-based moisturizer like Nivea or even Vaseline.

Soap and dry skin don't mix. But if you cannot forgo soap in the morning, this is what to do. Prepare a hot washcloth as above, then work your soap (preferably superfatted) into the cloth. Drape the soapy cloth over your face for about thirty seconds, and remove it with a single fast and light-handed wipe. Then, take a second unsoaped washcloth, drench with very hot tap water, and use it to pat off any remaining soap on the face. Pat yourself dry, again leaving a bead or two of water here and there, and moisturize as above.

If you have dry skin on your face, you shouldn't wash it more than twice daily; once a day is preferable. Your first washing should be upon awakening in the morning; the second should be at the end of the day's activities. But better than a second washing is the following Splash

Regimen: Fill the bathroom basin with cool to luke-warm water, splash the face, and pat dry. Then pat on Cetaphil Lotion, an over-the-counter preparation you can get at any well-stocked drugstore. Cetaphil cleans and lubricates without drying. In fact, in advanced cases of dryness it's a good substitute for soap.

16

Aging Skin: What to Do About It

Accepting your age with dignity makes you feel better and look better to the world. However, gracefully accepting that your days of being cute are over is no reason to let yourself go. This chapter will explain techniques that are used to make older skin look healthy and handsome. They'll even make your skin look younger. But do remember that true beauty in age rests on a foundation of physical health, mental equilibrium, and intelligent skin care. It isn't helped by vain attempts to pretend that you're younger than you are.

The Characteristics of Aging Skin

An aged appearance of the skin depends on conditions that vary for each of us. Obviously, your number of years on the earth plays a major part. But so do heredity, the amount of sun exposure you've endured through your life, and the condition of your hormones.

If you undertake to improve the appearance of your face, don't forget your hands and neck. To attend to one without taking care of the others is at least unaesthetic. Spotted, wrinkled hands hardly flatter a newly smoothed and moisturized face.

As the years pass, the skin becomes increasingly wrinkled, primarily from deterioration of elastic tissue and from dehydration. Although there are many things that you can do to make wrinkles look much better, there's nothing that stops them from appearing. Nor can you stop the lines and creases that gradually and permanently engrave your mental disposition onto the features of your face.

Other typical phenomena appear on the skin as the years advance. Little broken capillaries (senile angiomas), brown liver spots (senile lentigos), reddish crusted lesions (actinic keratoses), persistent blackheads (senile comedones), and an irreversible drooping of the flesh can all make for an unsightly appearance. Now here's the good news: Not only is every one of these conditions quite normal, but each—with the exception of drooping skin—can be wonderfully improved with the following suggestions. For drooping and sagging, I refer you to Chapter 7, "Cosmetic Surgery."

Environmental Protection

Skin that shows symptoms of aging has already gotten its lifetime allotment of sun exposure. This isn't to say that you can never walk hatless again, but it does mean that you are ill-advised to sunbathe, hike, play tennis, or do other things outdoors without wearing a sunscreen. As I've mentioned, my favorite sunscreen products contain PABA, which, as you'll recall, is the miracle ingredient in sunscreens like PabaGel, Presun, and Eclipse. It quite amazingly screens out the rays that cause skin cancer and dehydration. While younger people can better tolerate sun exposure, older people with wrinkles and spots should always protect their skin from the sun with PABA.

Since older skin is usually dry, I suggest looking at Chapter 15, "Dry Skin Regimens." Refer to the section on humidifying your environment for suggestions on how to prevent an overly dry home or office from robbing precious skin moisture.

What the Dermatologist Can Do for You

Working with a good dermatologist, you can completely eliminate many symptoms of aging skin. One of the best methods at the doctor's disposal is electronic desiccation. This is an extremely safe and almost painless procedure which employs a small electric needle. It can totally remove unsightly surface capillaries (senile angiomas) and liver spots (senile lentigos). The doctor touches the needle to the skin for a second or two, the current kills the cells in the affected area, and within a week or two the body sheds the dead cells and the angiomas and lentigos are gone. So safe is this electronic procedure that you can come back every six months or however often is necessary. But while you're attending to your face, don't overlook your hands, throat, or neck.

There's a do-it-yourself approach to liver spots, which employs Eldoquin, a bleaching cream. This is an OTC preparation that you can get at any well-stocked drugstore. It contains hydroquinone, a skin-bleaching agent that will bleach the brown color out of the lentigos, usually over a four-to-six-month period, without affecting the pigmentation of normal skin areas. About the only possible drawback to Eldoquin is the allergic reaction some people have to it. Rub a small amount onto your forearm and give yourself a sensitivity test. If nothing happens within twenty-four hours, then you probably won't have any allergic reaction. Rub it on several times daily and the spots will gradually fade. If you're going to be in the sun, be sure to use a PABA sunscreen in addition to the Eldoquin.

Perhaps the worst-looking of the aged skin lesions are the crusty reddish sores called actinic keratoses. When these lesions are biopsied, they show cellular disorganization, a precancerous condition. Many of them can be removed quite simply either by spot-freezing or by using a scalpel-like tool called a curette. With this latter method, the dermatologist simply scrapes the lesions off, and they rarely come back. It's as easy as that.

But sometimes curetting isn't a rigorous enough treatment. Then your dermatologist can prescribe Efudex, a nearly miraculous prescription drug that contains 5-fluorouracil. (This ingredient has the ability to destroy selectively only disorganized skin cells, leaving normal cells undisturbed. What's more, it can even perceive and act upon disorganized cells undetected by the naked eye.) The Efudex is applied once daily for a period of two to four weeks, during which time nothing seems to happen. Then a redness begins to appear on the affected areas. The medication is stopped, but the redness continues to get worse and worse. At this point many patients begin to hate their doctors or become convinced that the doctor has made the problem worse. The red affected areas begin to ooze and further red splotches appear on the face and hands where there had been no overt symptoms previously. During this period, I recommend application of soothing compresses dipped in a solution of one quart cool water mixed with two tablespoons of salt and a cup of skim milk (or two tablespoons of powdered milk). Some doctors prescribe fluorinated steroid creams to soothe the irritation, but steroids tend to thin the skin, and I think aging skin is already thin enough. Eventually the redness, oozing, and discomfort will decrease and then stop, fresh healthy skin will replace the crusty keratoses, and your appearance will be greatly improved.

If you have an important occasion coming up and you want to look your very best, you might consult with your dermatologist about a mini-peeling. This process will temporarily plump up wrinkles so as to give the illusion of smoother, more youthful skin. It's achieved by irritating the skin just enough to cause minor swelling and edema. Edema is the medical name for the fluid that irritated tissue will tend to collect temporarily. In my practice, I use trichloroacetic acid, the same chemical used for acne peelings. I just use less. The whole process is neither terribly irritating, nor particularly expensive. You should do it the day before the big event in order to give the skin time to get over the initial redness but not time for the minor swelling or edema to go down.

Rubifactants are organic irritants that do approximately the same thing. Instead of a mini-peeling, you might prepare a rubifactant mask for yourself, using the instructions in Chapter One, p. 5. Pineapples, papayas, strawberries, wintergreen, and pepper are all natural rubifactants. This won't smooth the face as much as the doctor's procedure, but it might be worth a try.

Estrogen Therapy

The female hormone estrogen makes skin smooth and soft; it gives it a radiant glow and helps maintain turgor. Many women take it orally after menopause, when the body's natural production declines. The results are often quite dramatic, and if that were all there were to it, then everybody would be taking estrogen pills.

But everything in life seems to be a trade-off. Estrogen therapy is the subject of a heated medical debate because many doctors think it either promotes or precipitates cancer. About every three months, medical opinion swings one way or the other. I personally think that some women benefit enormously from estrogen therapy, but I never prescribe it without detailing the risks and sending the woman to a gynecologist for Pap smears and a second opinion. If you're a forty-five-year-old woman with deteriorating skin, estrogen will make you look better.

But even without the estrogen, you're a possible candidate for cancer. What should you do? Get several medical opinions, assess the risk as best you can, and make a decision.

Epiabrasion

This is a do-it-yourself technique that's ideal for wrinkles and senile comedones. (See Chapter 8 for a more complete discussion of epiabrasion.) I confess that I never use the word "senile" to describe aging skin phenomena when I'm talking to patients. Senile only means old, but unfortunately it's weighted down with unflattering connotations. Old comedones, if you will, are just blackheads. They frequently affect the area between the eyes and the temples, and result from discolored oil plugs that are clogging up the openings of your pores.

Epiabrasion won't make wrinkles go away, but it will make them look much better. And it will also help open up and clean out those old blackheads. You can either buy an epiabrador (I think the Buf-Puf, available at good drugstores, is a fine product) or just use your washcloth. To epiabrade, you need only scrub the entire face (don't forget your hands and neck) vigorously every day. Give your skin time to adjust to daily scrubbing. Start out by doing it for less than a minute, then work up gradually until you can epiabrade comfortably for between two and four minutes. Don't be too vigorous, and if you overdo it, skip a day or two as needed.

Epiabrasion removes the top layers of the epidermis,

keeps the skin clean and stimulated, and promotes new cellular growth. It also provides mild irritation that keeps wrinkles attractively plumped and cushioned with a minimal and entirely safe level of edema. It's good for everybody, young or old, dry or oily, acne-prone or clear-skinned. You'll be amazed how many people will compliment your healthy vigorous complexion when you epiabrade regularly.

Remember, all these are temporary measures. They won't make wrinkles go away, but they will make them look much less obvious. Since aging skin usually tends to be dry, I suggest that you combine your daily epiabrasion ritual with a very oily soap. Oilatum, Alpha Keri, Tone, Basis, even Dove, Caress, or any of the cold-cream soaps do quite well. You might soften the soap by keeping a bit of water in your soap dish. They you'll be able to spread the softened soap onto your face like cold cream. Epiabrade for one to four minutes, wash with warm water, apply a thin layer of cold cream, and rub it in until it vanishes.

Epiabrade every day. If you do it in the morning, then follow the cold cream with your normal makeup or with an oil-based moisturizer. If you wait until evening, naturally you'll still need the moisturizer. Since the healthy ruddy glow tends to fade after a few hours, you'll look best if you epiabrade in the morning.

Moisturizing

Most women already use a moisturizer to combat natural dryness that comes with the passing years. The idea is to hydrate the face by washing with hot water and patting dry, then to lock in the moisture, which temporarily plumps up the wrinkles. To maximize the effect of your moisturizer, I recommend that you combine it half and half with one of the nonoily urea-based creams. Urea is an aquaphilic chemical, which means that it naturally attracts and holds moisture. The beauty of a urea moisturizer is that it tends to hold moisture without sealing the pores shut the way traditional oil-based moisturizers do.

Even though older women can tolerate pore-clogging moisturizers much better than their younger sisters, they can still benefit from the aquaphilic properties of urea. If you combine your favorite moisturizer with a urea cream like Aquacare, Aquacare/HP, or Carmol, you'll be getting the best of both worlds. If your skin is particularly dry, make your mixture heavier on the oil-based side.

Here are instructions for two intensive mini-moisturizing regimens. The first is made from heavy cream and Vaseline, combined in equal portions in a bowl. Since you don't have the emulsifiers to guarantee smooth combination, don't expect your mixture to be totally smooth. Combine as best you can, coat your face (and hands and neck) and leave the mixture on for half an hour. Wipe off with a moist warm towel, wash the face with a superfatted nondrying soap, pat dry, and apply your favorite moisturizer.

The second intensive mini-moisturizing regimen is essentially the same as the first, except that you first combine a handful of strawberries with the cream in a blender. Then mix the blended strawberries and cream with the Vaseline as above, and apply the same way. The strawberries are a natural rubifactant or mild stimulant. The treatment will not only give you an intensive moisturization but will also promote a mild irritation to further plump up wrinkles.

Finally, here's a regimen for maxi-moisturization that you can use twice a week at bedtime. Apply Vaseline all over the face, hands, and neck (or legs or anywhere else needed), and leave it on overnight. Don't cake it on, and rub it in well. In the morning, wipe it off with nondrying Cetaphil Lotion, and proceed with your usual makeup and moisturizing ritual. A night's worth of Vaseline is tremendously moisturizing; you'll wake up looking fantastic.

Summary: The Total Regimen

The following is a recapitulation of the suggestions in this chapter, plus a few final hints.

1. sun protection with PABA
2. regular visits to the dermatologist
3. estrogen hormone therapy (maybe)
4. epiabrasion once a day
5. moisturizing once a day (at least)
6. maxi-moisturization twice weekly
7. facial massage (at skin or cosmetic salons)
8. use oil-based (as opposed to water-based) makeup
9. eat more vitamins of the multiple one-a-day variety (aging skin particularly needs the help of Vitamin C in healing and Vitamin A to assure orderly cell maturation).

17

Large Pore Regimens

Do you know what's wrong with large pores? Nothing! The good Lord gave them to you, and medically speaking there's nothing bad about them. However, from a cosmetic standpoint, they are a source of numerous complaints. The goal of this chapter is to teach you ways to temporarily shrink your pore openings and gain a smoother complexion.

Most people think that pores are the surface openings of oil glands. The truth of the matter is that most pores are actually the surface openings of sweat glands. Sweat glands constitute the majority of the openings on the skin surface, and they coexist with varying numbers of oil glands and hair follicles. People with large pores don't necessarily have oily skin, unless of course they also have large or overstimulated oil glands.

Whether or not your pores are too large is a highly subjective matter. Since there is no medical liability in having large pores, they constitute a problem only if they look bad to you. You can study your skin in a 4X magnifying makeup mirror (available at drugstores), preferably at the end of the working day, when an average amount of oil production and dirt exposure has taken place. Enlarged pores are often found near the hairline, on the nose, and on the butterfly of the face. If you've never noticed your pores before, or really have to search to find enlarged varieties, then stop reading this chapter right here and move on. It is not my intention to add another worry—and a dubious one at that—to your life.

But if your pores seem unattractively large to you, then you can employ the following suggestions to make them look smaller. No one can actually make the pore openings shrink permanently. The size of your pores, like countless other individual aspects of your body, is genetically determined. The regimens that follow, like almost everything suggested in this book, will only make you look better temporarily. They won't permanently alter the structure of your body. And you have to keep doing them or your large-looking pores will quickly reappear.

Invigoration

Invigoration is a nice way of describing intentional inflammation of the skin. Continually inducing a mild degree of inflammation is not bad for your skin. On the contrary, it promotes good cell turnover, combats excessive oiliness that can lead to acne, and brings about

a minor amount of swelling that is actually quite flatter-
ing. Irritated tissue automatically attracts a fluid called
edema, which is a natural serum from your own blood.
Edema tends to plump up the tissue around the pore
openings, thereby making the pores appear smaller.

Regular epiabrasion, as described in Chapter 8, is
the best way to invigorate your skin. If you want a regimen that's more abrasive, substitute one of the acne
soaps—Acnaveen, Acne-Aid, Sulphur Soap—for your regular soap when epiabrading. Remember that since acne
soaps are usually quite drying, dry-skinned people must
properly moisturize the skin after washing. Chapter 15
has details on proper moisturization for dry skin. A rubifactant mask, such as the one described in Chapter 1,
will also invigorate the face.

Alternately, you can go to your dermatologist and ask
him to perform a mini-peeling. You will recall that this
is a brief, not-very-expensive process in which the doctor
paints an irritating chemical onto your face (I use varying strengths of trichloroacetic acid), then removes it
when several layers of cells have been burned away and
mild edema induced. The procedure gives you a ruddy
glow and the edema causes the plumping up of tissue
that swells pores partially shut. It's temporary and the
results last only a few weeks.

Another treatment your dermatologist might per-
scribe is chemabrasion, a technique often used to
smooth bad acne pits and scarring. Similar to a mini-
peeling, this process merely involves a larger amount of
irritating chemicals applied over a longer period of
time. The resulting plumping up of the tissue and ap-

parent diminution of the pores also lasts longer, sometimes up to six months.

Masks

The rubifactant mask mentioned above is recommended primarily for its irritating properties. But all masks have in common another, less fully understood property. It is thought that application of a mask somehow affects the electrical polarity of the skin. Whether or not this is true, masks certainly do tend to close up the pores. You can go to a drugstore or cosmetic counter, buy any pleasantly scented or packaged mask that strikes your fancy, and it will have a shrinking effect on your pores. Or you can also make a mask of your own from one of the recipes in Chapter 1. Here is another basic, no-frills mask that actually performs as well as any expensively packaged commercial product.

Dissolve a package of gelatin in a small amount of water and combine with the whites of two eggs. Take a sable brush and paint onto the face, leaving a comfortable margin around the eyes, mouth, and nose. Let dry for twenty minutes. Then rip the mask off as vigorously as you can. Splash the face with water, pat dry, and thoroughly rub in a thin layer of cold cream.

Astringents

Again for reasons not entirely clear to anyone, astringents tighten pores. Almost all of them are alcohol-based and are therefore quite drying. So if your oversized pores happen to accompany a dry skin problem, beware of frequent astringent application.

To make an impact on pores, you'll have to apply the astringent three to four times daily. This also makes it difficult to wear makeup. Neutrogena Acne Gel, Bonne Bell Ten-O-Six, Seba-Nil (which also comes in convenient towelettes), Wash 'n Dri, or, for that matter, witch hazel, rubbing alcohol, your favorite perfume, or a combination of alcohol and a few drops of perfume are all good astringents.

For an excellent astringent, ask your doctor for a prescription for 20 percent aluminum chloride tincture. Aluminum salts close up pores and are, in fact, a major ingredient in most of the widely marketed deodorants. This tincture is easy to apply and very effective, especially when added to a daily epiabrasion regimen with soap.

Creams and Ointments

Another approach that seems to work with some people is to supermoisturize the pores with a cream or ointment. Sensible application can plump them up attractively, but there is a danger of clogging shut neighboring oil glands (especially with ointment application) and precipitating an acne flare-up.

Jergens, Neutrogena, and Paquin make good hand creams that are ideal for this purpose. Dilute these or any good cold cream with a little water, then rub a moderate amount onto the large-pore area. I recommend that you alternate cream days with astringent days to avoid any pore clogging buildup on the skin.

The Super Regimen

This regimen would combine the approaches already outlined above into one concerted attack on your pores. It is irritating, so if you go all out, be cautious. Give your skin a chance to adapt. If undue irritation develops, discontinue the most irritating parts of the regimen.

1. Epiabrade every morning.
2. Wash with an acne soap such as Acne-Aid, Acnaveen, SAStid, Fostex, or Neutrogena Acne Soap.
3. Apply an astringent upon waking, at noon, at 4 P.M., and at bedtime, every other day.
4. Apply a cream once daily in the morning in between astringent days.
5. Apply your favorite mask three times weekly, and keep it on overnight.

There is an alternative to the above suggestions that will sometimes do the job just as well. It consists of simply covering the large pores with foundation makeup. About the only risk in this course of action is the possibility of an acne flare-up if your oil glands become clogged with cosmetics. Younger and usually more oily-skinned women must beware of makeup for this reason. But older women with drier skin might very well cover worrisome large pores with foundation and solve the problem to their satisfaction. Young or old, don't succumb to the temptation of using too much makeup. When excess makeup becomes lodged too deeply in the pores, it can accentuate them instead of covering them up.

18

Heads Up!
The Best Things to
Do for Your Hair

The very best thing for your hair, of course, is to find a good hairdresser. As for things you can do yourself, they all depend on what your hair problem is. It's beyond the scope of this book to discuss diseases of the scalp, so the following discussion will be limited to three common problems: thinning, dandruff, dry and oily-greasy hair.

Thinning Hair

Experience with this subject compels me to state right away that there is no such thing as a product that makes hair grow on your head. I shudder to think how many people each year are conned into spending good money on bogus hair-growth products. None of them work, so don't be fooled.

On the other hand, it is a medical fact that hair follicles hardly ever die. Even on a head that looks like the proverbial billiard ball, the follicles at least are alive. But whether or not they grow hair depends on hormone levels. Treatments such as scalp massages and vigorous vitamin rubs will only temporarily increase the blood supply on the scalp. Follicles are very receptive to hormones, but not to a mere increase of blood.

Advancing age—with its attendant hormonal changes —is the common cause of thinning hair. The hormone with the most adverse effect on the hair follicle is the "male" hormone androgen. Androgen is also produced in the ovaries and adrenals of the female body. After menopause, a woman's naturally high level of estrogen —the female sex hormone—begins to fall. Her hair follicles then find themselves undefended against the existing levels of androgen that had been tolerated without notice until then.

The result of all this has long been called "male pattern baldness." It consists of a retreat of the hairline coincidental with a thinning on the crown. In some women it can sometimes be stopped with systemic estrogen therapy.

I discussed the potential dangers of estrogen in the last chapter and cited the ongoing debate about whether or not it causes cancer. For now, let us say that estrogen is potentially dangerous. Systemic estrogen therapy, which involves taking a prescription pill called Premarin in the same way you might once have taken birth control pills, is as interesting as it is effective. Your body is fooled into a sort of premenopausal state during which you even have a period. This "period" is brought about when the Premarin is not taken—on every twenty-first day. (This induces a sympathetic withdrawal bleeding in the uterus.) The therapy also makes skin more moist and glowing and makes many formerly unhappy menopausal women feel better. Furthermore, eventually enough estrogen gets to the hair follicles to begin countering the effect of androgen. The therapy usually reverses postmenopausal hair loss within three months, but there is the element of danger (the possibility of cancer) that you should consider from the very beginning.

Before I leave the subject of estrogen, I'll mention that some doctors prescribe a lotion form of Premarin that's rubbed onto the scalp and is supposedly safer than the pills. I think it certainly must be safer, but I'm not at all sure that topical application can really get down into the subcutaneous regions that contain the roots of hair follicles. On the other hand, since it's not dangerous, if my doctor thought it would help, I would give it a try.

Now we all know that hair loss isn't limited to older people. Many doctors today feel that what's called a "subclinical" deficiency of iron can cause similar hair loss in younger women. The symptoms of acute iron deficiency include weakness, pallor, spooning of the nails, and hair loss. A subclinical deficiency is so mild that hardly any of the symptoms show. But since your

hair follicles are the most rapidly metabolizing structures in your body, deficiencies will affect them first.
Therefore, it is possible for you to be a young woman
leading a vigorous life, with so much energy that you
rarely feel tired (or do you?), and still be subclinically
iron deficient.

How do you find out if you are? The first thing is to
have your doctor give you the appropriate blood tests.
And if you had a recent blood test that showed nothing
unusual, it still doesn't mean you're in the clear. To
properly test for iron, you must get two tests—a serum
iron test and a serum total iron binding capacity test—
both of which require only a small sample of your blood.
Serum iron measures the quantity of iron in your blood-
stream; serum total iron binding capacity measures the
capacity of your blood to contain iron. In other words,
it is the measure of how much iron your blood potentially could contain. A normal ratio of iron is 1 to 5.
If your ratio is 1 to 7 or higher and you're losing your
hair, you might have a subclinical deficiency and probably would benefit from iron supplements.

Sometimes iron pills are prescribed in conjunction
with Premarin; sometimes the doctor suggests you take
them alone. The most typical iron pills are small and
green, require no prescription, and are available at any
well-stocked drugstore. They often cause quite normal
and harmless—if temporarily uncomfortable—side effects that include constipation, diarrhea, or black stools.
The black stools seem to provoke the most anxiety, but
they are an entirely normal side effect of iron pills, so
don't be frightened.

Despite the extreme sensitivity of hair follicles and their rapid metabolic rates, there seems to be a natural time lag between introduction of something into the system and noticeable effect on the hair. So as with Premarin, you'll have to be patient with iron therapy for at least a few months.

Other abnormalities besides iron deficiency may be thinning your hair prematurely. For example, a major cause of hair loss is malnutrition, a condition that can afflict a trendy diet faddist as easily as a peasant in the Third World. The problem with bizarre diets is twofold: First, they tend to eliminate whole blocks of necessary vitamins; and second, these diets are often subscribed to by people who haven't had a square meal in years. They leap from one bizarre diet to another, heedless of the damage it does to their bodies, at least until that damage becomes cosmetically obvious. Again, it's the high metabolic sensitivity of the hair follicles that makes them prone to trauma if a diet is unhealthful.

In addition to deficiencies in nutrition, physical shocks, illness, and many medicines can all precipitate hair loss. As a rule of thumb, if your hair is beginning to thin, avoid as many chemicals and medicines as possible. Even very common medications are associated with hair loss. These include cortisone, antithyroid drugs, L-Dopa (for Parkinson's disease), heparin (an anticoagulant), dilantin (an antiseizure medicine used in cases of epilepsy, brain tumors, etc.), borates (contained in boric acid as well as in certain mouth washes), aspirin (sad, but true), excessive amounts of Vitamin A, amphetamines, antibiotics, and certain poisonous anticancer drugs used in chemotherapy. Even the act of starting or stopping a course of birth control pills can sometimes trigger a bout of hair loss.

Any substantial shock to the system can very often be followed—in about three months—by partial or total hair loss. A diabetic coma, childbirth, any major illness, or being hit by a bus all qualify as major shocks.

But by far the most common cause of thinning hair among young persons who would not otherwise be expected to be balding is stress. It's indeed a cruel quirk of nature that, in addition to playing havoc with the complexion and disposition, a stressful existence will often make your hair fall out. In its most dramatic form, an experience of fright or horror can actually result in total (albeit delayed—and temporary) hair loss. People who have experiences like this will sometimes discover that their hair grows back completely white. Of course, the hair doesn't really turn white "overnight"; the process takes closer to three months.

As if hair weren't already imperiled enough, some people suffer from a nervous, stress-related condition called trichotilomania. This term describes people who sit distractedly, head cocked to one side, and methodically, unconsciously, twirl and yank out one strand of hair after another. They naturally get bald patches and are typically very resistant to the suggestion that they are pulling out their own hair. If you are one of these people and you're wondering what in the world to do, I suggest you explore hypnotherapy, probably the most successful solution that's yet been applied to trichotilomania.

So, then, a brief summary is in order. If your hair is thinning, there may well be nothing that you can do short of buying a wig or having a transplant. But you can easily determine whether or not your hair loss stems from one of the conditions just described. Have your blood levels of estrogen and iron checked by a doctor; maybe estrogen therapy would be ideal for you. Perhaps your hair problem stems from something about your life that you can change—diet, medication, or undue stress. Or perhaps from something that will pass, such as an illness or a profoundly shocking experience.

If you do have thin or thinning hair, the trick is to make it look thicker. First of all, thin hair always looks fuller when it's cut short. Moreover, the more you shampoo, the fuller your hair will look. It is not true that shampooing makes the hair fall out or that the strands on the bottom of the tub would still be on your head if you hadn't washed your hair. This is nonsense. The hair that's on the bottom of the tub would have fallen off the head anyway. In fact, the average rate of hair loss for a healthy person is between 100 and 200 hairs per day.

It is a good idea to shampoo daily because clean hair looks thicker. In addition, you can enhance the look of fullness with protein, which coats the hair shafts and gives an illusion of a thicker head of hair. There are all sorts of ways to get protein onto your hair. The most obvious is to use a shampoo that contains protein, like Protein 21 or Revlon's Milk and Honey. Or, you can use a protein conditioner immediately after you shampoo. There are also products called thickeners on the market that can give hair a needed dose of protein. Thickit and Pantene are both widely distributed and do the job well.

Here are some suggestions for do-it-yourself protein treatments. The major ingredients are raw egg whites and plain powdered gelatin. These things don't always mix perfectly, nor do they look as appetizing as a creamy and expensively processed cosmetic. Nevertheless, they do the job just as well. Remember that even though all manufacturers seem to want you to lather your hair twice (thereby consuming twice as much of their product), a single lathering will clean satisfactorily, won't unduly strip away natural hair coatings, and is more economical.

The first regimen would be to dissolve a small packet of gelatin in a little warm water just before shower time, put the dissolved mixture in a small cup, and carry it with you into the shower. Pour your normal amount of shampoo into the cup, mix with the gelatin, and shampoo, ending with a protein conditioner. The second regimen would be nearly identical, except for the addition of the whites of two eggs to the dissolved gelatin. Don't try to make up a home mixture of gelatin, egg whites, and shampoo in advance. This is an organic formula and without preservatives will go bad. Make it fresh before every shampoo.

Some people swear by beer shampoos, but since beer has a minimum of protein, there's not very much it can do for thinning hair. A better treatment would be to shampoo and condition, then comb in the whites of two eggs and a small amount of lemon juice (to prevent sticking) while the hair is still wet. Let the egg whites dry—overnight if possible—then comb out the hair.

A final word of advice: Buy a variety of protein conditioners and shampoos and avoid consecutive use of any one product. The human body seems to acclimate itself to medicines and cosmetics quickly, and variety usually enhances the effect of each product. A week in which you use seven different combinations of gelatin, egg whites, and protein cosmetics will result in a head of hair that looks fuller than if you shampooed the same way every day.

Dandruff

Dandruff can accompany thick, thin, oily, or dry hair. It isn't particular. The pathology of dandruff is closely related to that of its first cousin, psoriasis. Both conditions are the result of an accelerated turnover rate of skin cells. Dandruff is much less severe than psoriasis.

As you read this page, your entire skin surface is shedding worn-out cells while fresh cells are being manufactured below the surface. Normally, this is an invisible process. But when the turnover rate becomes too fast, the dead cells begin to build up. Dandruff flakes are just patches of dead skin cells.

Fortunately, there are plenty of excellent dandruff shampoos on the market. Zincon, Zetar, Sebulex, Selsun, Head & Shoulders, and Vanseb-T are all very good. To maximize the antidandruff effect of the shampoos, I would advise you to buy at least three different types, and use a different one each day. This will automatically increase the effectiveness of each shampoo, since it lessens the body's natural tendency to adjust to a medicine. If you have dandruff that resists the commercial shampoos, have your doctor prescribe a prescription shampoo.

Another time-honored and natural treatment for dandruff is sun exposure. Either sit bareheaded in the sun or use a sunlamp. Yes, go ahead and shine the sunlamp right onto the hair; it will help. Use the same regimen I gave you earlier for sunlamp use (see Chapter 8); start with five seconds per day and work up to a plateau of three to four minutes by increasing exposure by five seconds a day.

If you suffer from thinning hair and dandruff, then add protein to both your dandruff shampoo and your conditioner. If your hair is thick or normal, this isn't necessary. If you have overly dry or oily hair, combine the antidandruff suggestions with those below.

Excessive Dryness and Oiliness

Hair that's excessively dry should be washed as infrequently as possible. If you have dry hair, get in the habit of adding oil to your shampoo. You can often get all the oil you need just by adding a little olive oil to your favorite shampoo and by using a conditioner. Since many manufacturers produce separate formulas for dry, normal, and oily hair, always choose the dry hair formula.

If the hair is dry *and* thin, then you should still condition daily but limit shampoos to three times a week (or more or less depending on just how dry you are).

If your hair is dry and dandruffy, then add a conditioner to your dandruff shampoo, use it twice or three times a week, and use a conditioner alone on the other days.

For perpetually greasy hair, your aim is to strip away all the excess oil. The best way to do this is with an acne shampoo. Preparations like Pernox, PanOxyl, and Fostex are excellent degreasers, as is any castile shampoo.

For best results with the acne shampoos, I again urge you to buy a few different types; lather the first time with one, and the second time with another. If your hair is really oily, there is no need for conditioners. But you might also take some reconstituted lemon juice with you into the bathroom and rinse the hair with it in between latherings.

Aside from regular daily shampooing—and oily-headed people should definitely lather twice—there isn't much more you can do about oily hair. Stress can stimulate the oil glands, and since most of your hair follicles have a little oil gland attached, your already oily hair can become even oilier if you're under pressure.

If your hair is oily and dandruffy, then substitute the aforementioned dandruff shampoos—which also tend to be drying—for the acne shampoos. Again, alternate different brands of shampoos, and use a lemon juice rinse between latherings.

19

The Best Things to Do for Your Nails

Nature gave us nails in order to help us grasp things. But our civilized existence has largely diminished the need for nails. There are, in fact, many fellow human beings who have no nails at all—due to major infections, congenital diseases, severe psoriasis, and so forth —and still manage to get through life.

Here now are some fascinating facts about fingernails. To begin with, the nail itself is dead. It is produced by the skin tissue at the base of the nail, much as a hair is produced by its follicle. And like hair, there is nothing you can put directly onto the nail that will affect its growth at all.

Fingernails grow faster than toenails, but all nail growth is asynchronous. This means that every nail grows at its own rate. Your nails are also individually susceptible to the nail dangers itemized below. Each nail is unique unto itself, and it's often possible to have problems with some nails, while others remain unaffected.

The average growth rate of a human nail is between .1 and .12 millimeters per day. This fact was determined by an observant dermatologist from Iowa who spent over fifty years calibrating nail growth on a day-to-day basis. Other dermatologists have discovered that pregnancy, summer weather, and trauma (ranging from hammer blows to compulsive nail chewing) all tend to make nails grow faster.

Your general rate of nail growth is fastest during your second decade, and the rate declines thereafter. As the years pass, more and more calcium gathers in the nails. But calcium, contrary to popular myth, does not contribute to harder nails. Quite the contrary, it makes them brittle—as any older person will attest. Nor does ingestion of gelatin have any known affect on the nails. Nails, like hair, are almost pure protein, which is probably why the myth of the benefits of drinking gelatin (also pure protein) has persisted so long. The problem is that the gelatin you drink doesn't affect the skin from which the nail grows.

Nails are extremely porous and can absorb one hundred times as much water as an equal amount of skin. Nails soak up everything liquid, including nail polish. Nail preparations are tested so thoroughly that there's rarely a danger in their use. Occasionally quick-drying preparations can dehydrate and crack the nails, or residual polish can cause slight stains on the surface, but these are not frequent complaints.

What follows are four sections devoted to identifying and correcting the most common things that can go wrong with your nails.

Paronychia

When the skin at the base of your nail becomes infected the resulting swelling and inflammation is called paronychia. Not only does the inflammation make the skin tender and painful, but since nails grow out of this tissue, severe paronychia will produce dystrophy, or misshaping, of the nails. Dystrophic nails can be indented, spotted, spooned, split, and generally ugly.

People whose hands are wet all day are prime candidates for paronychia, also called barmaid's finger, since digits dipped in beer all day almost inevitably contract yeast infections. But anyone who works with lots of water—including housewives—is susceptible. Paronychia is so common that many people ignore it, thereby risking disfigurement of the nails.

The main thing to do for paronychia is to keep the hands as dry as possible. Decrease daily hand washings and buy fingercots, those little rubber caps that fit over the tip of each finger. Their only drawback is that some fingers become irritated by the fingercot rubber or become uncomfortably sweaty.

Another way to cure paronychia is with an OTC drug called Bacitracin. This is a "broad spectrum" antibiotic and is often effective in combating the infection and reducing tissue inflammation. Apply the Bacitracin several times a day. For very bad cases, you might consider having your doctor inject medicine directly into the inflamed tissue. This will counter the inflammation and help to avoid possible future nail disfigurement.

Whatever you do, it's imperative to dry up the skin on those hands now and to protect the inflamed fingers from future wetness.

Onycholysis

If your nails are separating from the tissue that lies beneath them (called the nail bed), then you've got onycholysis. It's a very common problem, but there is no regimen I can prescribe to cure it. The cure rests in accurately identifying and removing the cause, then allowing the nail to grow back.

Bacterial and fungal infections are the usual cause for separating nails. They resist topical antibiotics, so your doctor will have to give you prescription pills. Occasionally, people have allergic reactions to certain nail hardeners or to the glue used on artificial nails. These reactions lead to edema and swelling of the nail bed. (Edema, you will remember, is the name for the fluid that accompanies inflamed tissue.) Swelling and edema in the nail bed will dislodge the nail, thereby causing onycholysis.

Or the cause might be a photoallergic reaction resulting from the combination of some medicine you're taking and sun exposure. People tend to forget that nails are one of the most exposed parts of the body. It's quite common for a person to be taking a medication and have no noticeable reactions until he or she is exposed to bright sunshine. Oral diabetic medicines, blood pressure medicines, and especially Declomycin (prescribed for many acne sufferers) all have been connected with photoallergic reactions, specifically onycholysis. Sometimes thyroid disease and iron deficiency anemia will cause onycholysis also.

When nails begin to separate, many patients worry whether to pull them out, cut them back, or tape them down. What you should do is go directly to your doctor to determine the cause. He'll prescribe the appropriate treatment and the nails will heal themselves. It doesn't much matter what you do with the already damaged part of the nail. Please note that nails with onycholysis tend to be more susceptible to allergic reactions, so avoid nail cosmetics and artificial nails that might contain potentially allergenic adhesives.

Slow Growth and Brittleness

Nails that are flaky, prone to chip, full of white spots, slow growing, or pitted can result from any one or a combination of the following. Far too often it's a matter of a stress-related habit. Flick your nails all day, every day, for long enough and they'll look terrible. If it's not nerves, it might be a skin disease like psoriasis, a fungal infection, or poor blood circulation.

Again, if there's an obvious skin problem on the hands, have a doctor prescribe appropriate medicine. At home try supplementing your diet with iron pills. Be patient; nails are slow growers to start with, so a program of iron will take months before there's noticeable improvement. If the nails are unduly pitted or crumbly, try soaking them in a double-strength mixture of gelatin and water. Even though drinking gelatin won't do anything for nails, soaking them in it will cause temporary hardening and a promptly improved appearance. Alternately, you can buy combination hardener-lacquers at most drugstores. But remember, your first obligation is to eliminate any disease that may be causing the bad nails.

Here now is a do-it-yourself nail-hardening recipe, but it does, however, require a doctor's prescription. Your pharmacist will have to prepare it specially, but I include the formula in case your doctor isn't familiar with it. A pharmacist showed it to me, and I think it's very good, particularly since the nails can be painted with polish after treatment. The concoction is made from 15 percent camomile powder, 35 percent witch hazel, and 50 percent Formalin (a preservative), to which a dash of garlic and a drop of brilliant green color are added. It should be applied three times a week. Instead of making a special visit, you might jot the formula down, or mark this page, then ask your doctor or gynecologist for the prescription the next time you have an appointment. Caution: some people find this preparation irritating. If that includes you, discontinue using it.

Discolored Nails

In many ways, discoloration is the least serious thing that can happen to your nails. Often it's nothing more than the residue of colored nail polish that has been absorbed into the porous nail. If it bothers you, you can carefully scrape it off with a sharp knife.

Sometimes nails discolor for systemic reasons. For example: If you're deficient in Vitamin B_{12}, your nails can blacken; if you're taking certain antimalarial drugs, blue-brown lines can appear on the nails; phenolphthalein, a chemical found in both laxatives and some inexpensive wines, can cause dark gray spots; arsenic causes white bands; and so forth. These are all symptoms your doctor can recognize and treat.

Perhaps the most frequent discoloration of the nails is caused by a simple bruise. If the nail is struck with or against something hard, the nail bed can bleed and the blood can become trapped beneath the nail itself. This trapped blood soaks into the porous nail and stays there until the nail grows out.

Some chemicals can stain the nails. Photographic-developing chemicals often blacken them. The resorcin in certain nail lacquers sometimes causes red-black discolorations. These can be corrected merely by discontinuing exposure.

But there is one nail discoloration that bodes very ill for you indeed. At first, it can look like just another bruise on the nail. But unlike a bruise, it won't grow out. Instead it simply sits there and spreads. Far from being a bruise, this is a symptom of malignant melanoma, the only life-threatening variety of skin cancer. It's very rare, but terribly dangerous. So if you've got a nail bruise that hasn't moved in weeks, put this book down right now and call the doctor.

20

Acne

Acne is a disease of the oil glands that plagues almost as many adults as teenagers. Now let's see how it works. The job of the oil glands in your skin is to produce sebaceous oil. This oil is a benign substance that acts as a natural moisturizer. In normal quantities and by itself it does not cause acne. However, when the hormone balance of the body is altered—specifically, when the amount of androgen and androgenlike hormones increase—oil glands can and usually do become over-stimulated. Occasionally, the gland itself becomes enlarged and oil production automatically increases.

The excess oil gathers beneath and above the skin surface. Often, in spite of regular washing, oil begins to clog the openings of oil glands, hair follicles, and pores. This is where the problem begins, because within those pores, follicles, and glands live a host of normal skin bacteria. These bacteria metabolize the skin oil and produce slightly irritating by-products. (Bacteria, incidentally, have an amazing capacity to alter oils. They are even used as part of the latest technology in degrading offshore oil spills!)

If the chemically altered sebaceous oil becomes trapped within an oil-clogged pore, it begins to irritate the surrounding tissue. Inflammation results, the body sends a host of white blood cells in an attempt to engulf the foreign substance, and presto, you've got a pimple. A combination of oil and white blood cells form the pussy contents, and a semihardened oil plug spanning the entrance to the skin opening forms the pimple's head.

Acne eruptions include whiteheads, blackheads, pustules, and cysts. They all result from excessive oil that clogs up skin openings and traps the irritating products of normal bacterial metabolism. The top of a whitehead is simply a visible oil plug; a blackhead is a pigmented or dirty plug. Cysts and pustules often result from irritation below the skin surface, and they don't always have obvious heads.

Why do most pimples show up on the face and back? Because that's where you find a large concentration of oil glands. Can you get pimples elsewhere? Yes, indeed, they can show up wherever an oil gland becomes overstimulated and produces enough oil to clog itself. Compared to the face, arms, buttocks, legs, and so forth have very few oil glands. But they do have some, and the glands can become overstimulated—with the same effects seen much more frequently on the face.

Substances that cause pimples are called "acnegenic."

But something is acnegenic only to the extent that it stimulates the oil glands to produce excess oil. The biggest stimulant actually isn't a substance at all—I refer to stress and worry. Sad to say, an anxiety-ridden life very often causes pimples. The reason is that stress is believed to stimulate the adrenals, which in turn secrete excessive amounts of cortisone and androgen. Of course, we all have individual susceptibilities to hormones, but current medical thinking has it that high stress-induced levels of androgen overstimulate the oil glands, thereby setting the stage for acne.

Many medicines act on oil glands too, and they either trigger acne flares or make existing problems worse. Common examples include the following:

Cortisone (prescribed for arthritis, rashes, inflammation, and so forth)
INH (an anti-TB drug)
Expectorants that contain iodine (these are medicines that make you spit or loosen phlegm; they're often used for asthma patients)
Certain birth control pills (usually of the progesterone type)
Dilantin (a medicine for seizures stemming from epilepsy, brain tumors, and numerous other medical problems)

Sometimes your diet is an unsuspected cause of acne. But I hope you're not among the uninformed who still think that chocolate, french fries, or sugar cause acne. None of these substances has any effect on your hormones. And, I repeat, hormones are what stimulate the oil glands. The real culprits are foods high in iodides, bromides, and androgen. Unfortunately, this includes many health foods, such as wheat germ, kelp, shellfish, and peanuts. Also very androgenic are organ meats (kidney, liver) and Vitamin E (whose molecular structure is similar to androgen).

The Various Approaches to Treating Acne

First we'll talk about traditional topical therapy. The aim of this approach is to unplug the pimples, clean out the pus, and dry up as much oil as possible. This does not prevent acne; it just dries up what's already there. It's preventative only to the extent that drying medicines may degrease and unclog the skin before further irritation has a chance to develop.

All acne medicines, be they prescription or over-the-counter, contain variants of the following chemicals: alcohol (for drying); salicylic acid (a peeling agent); sulphur (for peeling and mild antibacterial effect); and resorcin (also a peeling agent). None of these chemicals, nor their close chemical relatives, will affect hormone levels or the rate of oil secretion. Still, there are excellent products that promote needed drying and peeling that together counter the oiliness. Brand names I consider very good include: Fostex, Clearasil, Rezamid, Vanoxide, Sulfacet, Komed, Klaron, and Postacne. There are doubtless a number of other equally effective products, but these I know to be good.

A more direct approach to getting rid of acne would be hormonal. But this is a course fraught with peril.

Eunuchs, as you may or may not know, never have acne problems because the absence of testes removes the source of androgen. Fortunately, there are other ways to counter androgen in the system, particularly for women. I refer to estrogen therapy, during which women take daily pills containing the female sex hormone estrogen. These pills do wonderful things for your hair and your complexion while they combat androgen. But as I have noted, estrogen therapy is thought in some medical circles to induce cancer. This is by no means a proven fact, and there are a large number of women on estrogen therapy of one sort or another. But there is an element of risk. Sometimes just a switch of birth control pills (to an estrogen type) is enough to counter acnegenic androgen. Ask your gynecologist if you think your pill might be giving you acne.

The third main approach to acne involves antibiotics. This type of therapy employs either of two widely used and widely publicized drugs: tetracycline and erythromycin. The idea behind antibiotic therapy is either to kill the bacteria or to alter their metabolic processes in such a way that the altered skin oil won't be irritating. These drugs have been in use for years and they work well. But the patient must be prepared to take significant doses for an extended period of time. If you're the type of person who is leery of pills on general principle, maybe you should try something else. When the pills don't work, it's usually because the patient stopped taking them too soon.

There are other drawbacks to antibiotic acne medicines. Tetracycline, for instance, has a strong chemical affinity to calcium. This means that once in your system, the drug can be easily sidetracked by any calcium that happens to cross its path. If it encounters calcium, it will bind to it and never get to the skin surface or to the bacteria it's supposed to combat. I've heard many patients adamantly maintain that tetracycline doesn't work, and that they know it for a fact since they've been taking it for three years. It usually turns out they've been taking it at mealtime. This is a forgivable temptation, since the drug tends to upset the stomach and food masks the discomfort. But calcium in the diet sidetracks the drug before it has a chance to work. You should take tetracycline on an empty stomach either one hour before or two hours after mealtime.

Tetracycline is considerably more effective than erythromycin, which is why it's the preferred drug for most acne sufferers. But it has other unpleasant side effects. Since it suppresses bacteria that normally suppress yeast, you run a higher chance of developing pesky yeast infections and vaginitis. If you know you're prone to vaginitis, be sure to tell your doctor before he prescribes anything. Because of its strong calcium-binding properties, tetracycline can't be given to children under sixteen, for there is a strong possibility that their teeth will develop unappetizing greenish-brownish stains. It's never given to pregnant women either, lest it stain the teeth of the developing fetus.

Erythromycin has fewer side effects, but it is not as effective. Stomach upset and vaginitis can result from the drug, but it's safe for children and supposedly for pregnant women too. Personally I don't believe pregnant women should take any medication. But, fortunately, their skin is usually quite lovely anyway.

What's New?

The newest, hottest thing in acne therapy is topical antibiotics. Although as of this writing the treatment is not yet FDA-approved, it holds out hope to people who want the antibacterial effects of antibiotics but don't want to take quantities of pills. Basically, this medication contains erythromycin (or another drug called Cleocin) in a drying base. It is applied daily and I understand the results are terrific. The prescription, however, can be expensive.

Another relatively new treatment is topically applied Vitamin A acid. It's called RETIN-A, and its effect is to alter the linings of oil glands so that oil secretion decreases. Again, this is strictly prescription stuff and is very strong medicine. It is typical in RETIN-A treatment for the acne to get worse before it gets better. You'll need patience and confidence in your doctor. It really does work, however, especially on acne that's dominated by blackheads and whiteheads.

What to Do If You Have Acne

The most important thing to do if you have recurrent acne is to go to the dermatologist at least once. You may think your condition is not bad enough to warrant a doctor bill, but I believe that money spent on your physical appearance is never wasted. Life is short and the "pursuit of happiness" is written right into the Declaration of Independence!

It is important to take a good look at your own life to see if you're causing the acne yourself. Do you live in a continual atmosphere of stress? Are you taking acnegenic medicines or eating acnegenic foods? Or are you clogging your own pores with acnegenic Vitamin E oils or heavy cosmetics? Cosmetics are so often the cause of acne that a new term, "acne cosmetica," has entered medical parlance. Occlusive (pore clogging) cosmetics can seal oil and bacteria beneath the skin just as easily as excess oiliness can. If you're at all acne-prone, you should at least avoid oil-based cosmetics in favor of less occlusive water-based formulas. And the fewer cosmetics you put on your face, the less chance of occlusion. (For more details on makeup, see Chapter 6.)

Here now are a selection of important elements for an antiacne skin regimen. You can use all of them or just some of them, depending on the severity of your acne problem.

Epiabrade Daily: Vigorous washing of the face helps keep pores open and free of excess oil. It promotes minor beneficial peeling and makes you look terrific. Chapter 8 has more details on epiabrasion, but here I'll simply repeat that it involves little more than scrubbing the face thoroughly. You can use either a specially designed epiabrador or your washcloth.

Use a Drying Soap: Neutrogena, Neutrogena Acne, Sulphur Soap, SAStid, Fostex, or plain old Ivory are all good choices. If you want to step up your attack, then use one of the acne soaps that contain little scrub granules like Pernox Scrub, Ionax Scrub, Komex, or Brāsivol. Be careful, these are purposely abrasive, so don't scrub yourself too much. But the point is to strip away excess grease and open up clogged pores, and sometimes granules are ideal for this.

Squeeze Pimples Carefully but Regularly: Yes, go ahead and do it; it's part of the treatment. The sooner you open up the pimple and clean it out, the sooner you'll put an end to the irritation stemming from trapped bacteria and oils. Cosmetologists can clean out your face for you or you can do it yourself. If you choose to do your own face, it's very helpful to have a comedo extractor, that handy little instrument described on p. 65 that looks like a dentist's tool. The procedure is to nick the top of the pimple (called deroofing), cover the nick with the spoon hole, and press from the side. It's not a difficult technique, and anyone can get the hang of it. Squeezing your own pimples is emphatically recommended with one exception: beware of the "triangle of death." This is the area of forehead just above the nose and the portions of the cheeks directly adjoining the nose. An infection here can lead to fatal complications if it drains into one of the sinus cavities.

Get Some Sun: Acne typically responds wonderfully to sun exposure, probably because of the beneficial peeling induced by the sun and the resultant removal of oil plugs. (Chapter 9 has details on how to take a sun-bath.)

Use a Drying Shampoo: Oiliness can be a problem on the hair as well as on the face. And excessively oily hair often causes pomade acne, breakouts at the hairline. If you're designing a program to counter oily skin, consider using a shampoo like Pernox, PanOxyl, Zetar, or Zincon.

Buy OTC Acne Medicine: These products help dry up existing acne eruptions and should be part of your personal program. Some that I like are Rezamid, Komed, Sulfacet, Clearasil, and Fostex. Don't smear your entire face; just treat the affected areas.

Beware of Cosmetics: Don't make acne worse by caking your face with pore-clogging cosmetics. If you want to cover a disaster spot, I recommend Liquimat. This has a water-based formula, it covers well, and contains medicine. Your pharmacist can even color-blend the stuff to match your complexion. It's my favorite cosmetic.

The following chart was published in a 1976 issue of *Cutis* magazine. It gives the results of an experiment conducted by Dr. James Fulton, whose purpose was to rate—on a scale of 0 to 5—the "comedogenicity" (tendency to cause pimples) of a variety of widely used cosmetics, acne preparations, lanolins, surfactants (the lubricating substances in makeup), and so forth. The experimenter used rabbit ears in lieu of young female cheeks, and here are his results. Zero is a good score; 5 is the worst possible.

COSMETICS	GRADING
Elizabeth Arden—Illusion Foundation	2
Ardena Velva Cream Mask	1
Ardena Moisture Oil	4
Yardley—Shine Stopper	2
Revlon—Eterna 27	3
Natural Wonder Alive & Free	2
Natural Wonder Anti-Acne Spot Cover	4
Ultima II Transparent Tawny Tint	5
Ultima II Transparent Wrinkle Cream	3
Ultima II Under Make-Up Moisture Lotion	3
Marcelle—Make-up base for oily skin	2
Avon—Ultra-Cover	3
Clear Skin Liquid Make-up	2
Covergirl—Super Sheer	3
Pond's—Moisture Cream	3
Allercreme—Petal Lotion	3
Matte Finish	4
Satin Finish	5
Velvet Finish	3
Reflecta	4
Merle Norman—Tahitian Tan	3
Love's—A Little Cover	3
Almay—Liquid Make-Up	2
Tint Naturel	3
Lancome—Maquimat	3
Fabergé—Xanda	2
Germaine Monteil—Moisture Make-Up	4

Clinique—Balanced Moisture Make-Up	4
Continuous Coverage	4
Noxzema Skin Cream	3

ACNE PREPARATIONS	GRADING
Contrablem	3
PanOxyl	1
Transact	2
Clearasil	3
Liquimat without sulfur	4
Liquimat with sulfur	3

LANOLINS	GRADING
Anhydrous Lanolin	2
Amberlate P	3
Lanolin Absorptive Base	2
Amberlate LFA	2
Sterolan	3
Acetol	4
Acetulan	4
Waxolan	1
Ethoxylated Lanolin	3
Lantrol	2
Isopropylan-50	3
Amerchol	2
Lanosterin	3
Liquid Lanolin	3
Lanogene	3

SURFACTANTS AND EMULSIFIERS	GRADING
Isopropyl Myristate (5%)	3
Isopropyl Myristate (100%)	5
Myristyl Myristate	4

Ascorbyl Palmitate	2
Sodium Lauryl Sulfate (1%)	3
Sodium Lauryl Sulfate (5%)	4
Tween 20	2
Brig 30 (1%)	1
Cetyl Alcohol	1
Stearyl Alcohol	1
Stearic Acid	2
Glycerol Monostearate	1
Isopropyl Isostearate	5
Butyl Stearate (5%)	3
Butyl Stearate (100%)	5
Robane	2
Hexadecyl Alcohol	5

MISCELLANEOUS	GRADING
Crude Coal Tar 1%	5
Hydrophilic Ointment	3
Candelilla Wax	1
Sulfur (ppt) 10% in alcohol gel	2
Sulfidal® 10% in alcohol gel	1
Titanium Dioxide	0
Glycerin	0
Castor Oil	1
Iron Oxide pigments	0
Propylene Glycol	0
Mineral Oil (various preparations)	0–2
Propyl gallate	2
Methyl Paraben	0
Propylene glycol	0
Butylene glycol	2
Hexylene glycol	3
Polyethylene glycol 300	3

21

Black and Beautiful

Skin is pigmented by a protein called melanin, produced in everybody's skin by structures called melanocytes. Occasionally, black people have a bit more melanin, but having a little more is not what makes the skin dark. Rather, skin coloration depends on how the little packages of melanin are dispersed.

The following illustration should make this clear: We take two glasses of water (representing two skin cells) and add a drop of India ink to each. If we leave the first unmixed and undispersed, the water will remain predominantly clear. However, if we mix up the ink and water in the other glass, it will appear considerably darker than the mixture in the first glass. The difference in color results from dispersion, not from unequal amounts of pigmenting substances. In human beings, pigmentation dispersion is genetically determined. Whether your skin is onyx, caramel, chocolate, beige, or pale white depends on the degree to which the genes governing dispersion express themselves.

The biggest benefit of dark skin is its natural resistance to damaging sunlight. A summer tan represents the efforts of white skin to achieve the same level of protection that dark skin already enjoys. Of course black people get sunburned, but to a lesser degree than do whites. The natural melanin dispersion in black skin also retards wrinkling and slows sun-induced disintegration of elastin. You'll recall that the result of damaged elastin is drooping, sagging flesh. Best of all, dark pigmentation significantly reduces the incidence of skin cancer.

But black skin is subject to a variety of problems, and the following sections deal with the most common of these.

Keloidal Scarring

Keloids are thick unsightly scars, and almost anything —a pimple, a shaving nick, or an incision for cosmetic surgery—can cause them. Not everybody gets keloidal reactions, but while about 1 percent of white people get keloids, the percentage is substantially higher among blacks.

Keloids present a unique problem, since removing them surgically only results in more keloids. Many of them are permanently disfiguring. But others can be successfully removed or substantially diminished by injecting steroids directly into the scar. For this sort of treatment, consult a dermatologist.

Every black person old enough to read this book should have some idea of her or his own tendency toward keloid reactions. Some people have much less of a problem. Whatever you do, be extremely cautious about any cosmetic surgery. Silicone implantation, surgical removal of stretch marks, face-lifts, eye debagging, and especially dermabrasion or chemabrasion can all be seriously disfiguring if you're prone to keloids. It's a topic you must discuss thoroughly with your doctor before he touches your skin. This is very important and cannot be stressed too much.

People who are very prone to keloids sometimes suffer from acne keloidalis. They get a little keloid on every acne eruption, which can look terrible. The treatment is vigorous acne therapy, details of which are given a little later on in this chapter. Under no circumstances should people with this condition undergo either chemabrasion or dermabrasion, which could easily transform the face into one massive keloid.

Postinflammatory Hypopigmentation and Hyperpigmentation

These high-sounding words refer to the tendency of black skin either to lighten or darken after acute inflammation resulting from psoriasis, rashes, burns, bad acne, and so forth. Again, the problem is by no means limited to dark skin; it's just more prevalent and noticeable there.

With hypopigmentation (lightening), almost nothing can be done. In cases of hyperpigmentation (darkening), you can apply a cream that contains a bleaching agent called hydroquinone. Eldoquin and Esoterica are two widely respected OTC preparations for hyper-pigmentation. Use them (or anything that contains hydroquinone) together with a sunscreen (get one that contains PABA, like Presun, Eclipse, PabaGel, etc.), as sun exposure makes hyperpigmentation worse.

If you suffer from acne, be aware that the chemical resorcin, which is widely found in acne medications, can darken black skin. Read the label before you purchase any acne medicine and be sure that it contains neither resorcin, nor any chemical whose name seems derived from the same word stem. Vanoxide, Komed, and Persa-Gel are three good acne medications that don't contain resorcin.

Acne

Almost everybody has some trouble with acne at some point in life, but black people face a few extra problems. Sometimes severe acne can result in acne keloidalis. Sometimes the acne will constitute an inflammation severe enough to induce hyperpigmentation. And if neither of those conditions occur, then sometimes the acne medicine itself will be irritating enough to provoke an unwanted reaction. So you're walking a tightrope between the acne inflammation itself and the potential inflammation that might be caused by acne medicines.

Still, the bulk of the advice in Chapter 20 is applicable to black and white skin alike. Of course, you should avoid any medicine with resorcin. But I recommend a vigorous program of topical therapy designed to degrease the skin and avert the excess oiliness that triggers acne. Use an acne soap like Sulphur Soap, SAS-tid, or Acnaveen, possibly in combination with an acne shampoo like Pernox, PanOxyl, or Danex. Shampoo once daily, and wash the face at least three times a day. Avoid greasy pomades, as they contribute to pore-clogging oiliness on the face. The cleaner and more grease-free you keep the face, the less acne you'll have to contend with.

If hyperpigmentation isn't a problem, consider using a sunlamp. A dark complexion means you can use the lamp longer than is recommended for light skins. Your melanin dispersion protects you to the point where you should be able to safely start out with thirty seconds' exposure, and work up via ten-second increments to a daily plateau of about four minutes. It should go without saying that if you start to burn, reduce the dosage. Don't skip a day. Be sure to move the face slowly from side to side and up and down, so as to insure even exposure. Sunlight and sunlamps have the same salutary affect on dark-skinned acne as on light-skinned acne. To be sure, you'll tan darker, but the color will be even and the acne should be improved.

Antibiotic acne therapy is also very effective for dark skin. This involves prescription pills (usually tetracycline) and involves no particular risks for dark skin. Details are in Chapter 20, "Acne."

Ingrown Hair

This is a problem often—though not always—found in those areas where you shave. When cut flush with the skin surface, the microscopic spiraling of the hair can sometimes cause it to grow back into the skin. This causes inflammation, shaving bumps, and often keloids.

It's a tough problem, and about the only thing you can do about it is mix an anti-inflammatory steroid cream with your shaving cream, then apply the cream alone after shaving. However, this will *not* stop the hair from growing inward. You can hope that daily usage will combat possible inflammation, thereby alleviating the problem somewhat. Steroid creams are prescription items that require a visit to the doctor. Alternately, you can go to any drugstore and buy Bacitracin, an OTC wide-spectrum antibiotic that may possibly help. You might want to experiment with it in lieu of the steroid creams and see if it works for you.

Hot Comb Alopecia

This term applies to hair loss that often plagues people who straighten their hair with hot oils. The most common problem areas are on the sides of the head, usually just above the ears.

The trouble with hot oils is that they tend to travel down the entire length of the hair shaft and enter into the follicle. If they're hot enough, they can fry the hair root, resulting in hair loss that is not always immediately noticeable. Sometimes months can pass before the hair actually falls out.

The solution rests laregly on your own ingenuity. It's the hot oil getting onto the scalp that's causing the problem, so if you can figure out a way to avoid that, you've got it licked.

Ashy Gray Dermatitus

Many black women come to me saying, "Doctor, my skin is turning white and ashy!" It's a common problem, especially on the face and upper trunk. Doctors call it "pityriasis alba," but giving it a name is not the same as fully understanding it.

It's my opinion that this condition is just a result of excessive dryness. I refer you to the dry skin regimens in Chapter 15 and suggest that you try some of the superhydration regimens.

Tinea Versicolor

This is a surface fungus whose excretory by-products constitute an excellent sunscreen. As long as your skin is out of the sun, you may never even know that you're host to tinea versicolor. But spend a few hours at the beach, and an irregular blotchiness appears. This blotchiness results from the irregular areas affected by the fungal by-products and, therefore, untanned by the sun.

It can look awful, but don't be frightened since the cure—the same no matter what your color—is quite simple. It consists of washing with Stiefel Anti-Fungal Soap, which kills the fungus, removes the by-products, and allows resumption of even tanning. If the affected area is small, you might want to try Tinactin, another good

OTC product, but too expensive if you need daily applications over a large area of the body.

I want to close this chapter by noting the recent and dramatic improvement in the quality of cosmetics for black women. And while on the subject of cosmetics, you should know that most good pharmacies can color-tint things like acne medicines as well as makeup to match your complexion. It's easy and inexpensive, and you don't have to buy expensive prescriptions to qualify for the service. Many women are either too shy or don't know that the service exists. Even inexpensive products like Klaron and Fostril can be taken out of the package, color-blended, and handed right back to you for a modest charge.

22

Lips

The skin on your lips is significantly different from the rest of your skin. Epidermal cells from the lips, when seen under a microscope, appear flattened. This makes the skin on your lips thinner and more sensitive both to changes in your interior chemistry and to influences in the environment.

Like the rest of the skin, lips are an interface between you and the physical world. Besides sun and weather, they're often exposed to exotic foodstuffs and a substantial variety of chemicals in today's health and beauty aids. For all this, the lips are amazingly durable. The lower lip, however, suffers a disproportionate share of lip problems, due primarily to the fact that it gets the most sun exposure.

The following are seven of the most common prob-

lems that affect lips, along with regimens and suggestions to correct each one.

Chapping

Lips get chapped when they become excessively dry.
Usually this dryness is caused by some environmental
factors like cold weather, undue exposure to strong
winds or desert sun, or too much time in centrally
heated houses (notorious for dehydrating the skin).

If your lips are chapping for reasons like this, you can
moisturize them with an ointment and wait for your
world to humidify. Chapstick is a familiar and excellent
standby, as is Vaseline, Crisco, or even things like Wesson oil, butter, or plain lipstick. Alternatively, you can
cover the lips with a small amount of baby oil, then
apply a cream lipstick. Frequent application is required
no matter what you use. The purpose of all these methods is to create an occlusive shield over the lips that will
prevent further dehydration.

Another approach is to humidify your environment.
This can be done with a home humidifier, or more
simply by just setting out shallow tubs of water around
the house. The tubs will evaporate naturally and moisturize the air. However, a humidified home won't be
much help if you spend eight hours a day in a dry
office. Whatever you do, beware of getting too many
drying chemicals on the lips. Things like soap, astringents, mouthwash, toothpaste, nail polish (you'd be
surprised what people get on their lips) are all very drying, so be careful.

Alternately, you might be causing your chapping problem all by yourself. I refer to compulsive lip licking. I
think everybody's mother has told them at some point
not to lick chapped lips. The reason, whether Mother
knew it or not, is that constant wetting leads to constant
evaporation. That's why doctors use wet compresses to
dry up oozy wounds. Quite often I see patients with
terrible chapping problems who tell me, between licking
their lips, that they've just moved into the city or just
gotten a big new job. They can't understand how the
chapping problem started up, since they've never been
bothered before.

It's obvious that stress and anxiety have resulted in
their nervous lip-licking habit that is chapping the lips.
And a whole barrel of Chapstick won't really help if
one doesn't get to the anxiety at the bottom of things.
Sometimes lip licking is a manifestation of infinitely
complicated psychological problems that can require
years of psychotherapy. And sometimes it becomes an
unconscious habit that responds well to hypnotherapy.
Personally, I have a lot of faith in hypnotherapy. How
do you find a hypnotherapist? Call your local county
medical society, and ask them to recommend a doctor
who practices it in your area.

Perleche

Here's another very common lip complaint most often—but not exclusively—seen in children and old folks.
It's characterized by cracking of the lips at the fissures
in the corners of the mouth and is often accompanied

by irritation on the skin just below the corners. It feels uncomfortable and doesn't look very attractive.

Perleche is caused quite simply by excessive salivation. The saliva drips out and irritates the lip corners and surrounding skin. In children, this is nothing more than a natural tendency to drool. In old folks, it sometimes stems from a neurological problem or improperly fitted dentures. Dentures can slightly alter the crucial angle of the mouth, and when this happens nothing ever seems exactly right again. Even if the alteration is unnoticeable to the wearer, it might be enough to cause slight drooling and eventually perleche.

On the other hand, there are people who oversalivate for medical reasons. If this applies to you, my advice is to go to a doctor. There are medicines to treat this condition. In the meantime, you can use a good thick lipstick or ointment to protect the lip corners from the saliva. And Bacitracin, a dependable OTC antibiotic ointment, when rubbed on the inflamed skin surrounding the mouth will help prevent secondary infection.

Pimples on the Lip Border

Certain people are prone to pimples right on the edge of the lip. This is a problem only because normal acne medications are too irritating for sensitive lip tissue. My suggestion is to dip a toothpick into a quality acne medication like Klaron or Vanoxide and touch it to the top of the pimple. Don't get any on your lips. The medication will induce a mild peeling that will eventually deroof the pimple and eliminate it.

Sunburn

It's very common to go out in the sun for the first time, get only the mildest touch of color, and still have your lower lip swell up. Even though the rest of you didn't get burned, your lip did. Why? Because the skin of the lips lacks melanin, the substance that pigments the skin and protects it from the sun.

Everybody talks about protecting their skin from the sun, then promptly forgets about the lips. Lips should always be protected, but they pose some unique problems. Use of PABA sunscreens would be great, but they taste terrible and inevitably tend to get licked off. Sun blockers like zinc oxide or Lassar's paste are even better, but you'll walk around looking like a clown.

Perhaps you haven't heard about Lassar's paste, which is essentially zinc oxide mixed with a tacky paste. Light from the sun can't penetrate a sun blocker, but the problem is to make it cosmetically acceptable. You might try buying a dark colored lipstick, mashing it together with Lassar's paste, and using the new combination whenever you're in the sun. Alternatively, you can ask your pharmacist to color-blend the Lassar's paste for you. After a day of sun exposure be sure to moisturize the lips with Vaseline or Aquaphore before you go to bed.

Lesions on the Lips

A lifetime of sun exposure on unprotected lips can cause actinic keratoses. These are ugly patches of disorganized skin cells that can occur anywhere on the sun-exposed skin of older people. This isn't quite skin cancer, but it is certainly a precancerous condition. The keratoses are also ugly, reddish, bumpy, and sometimes crusted.

If neglected, these actinic keratoses can develop into squamous cell carcinoma, a type of skin cancer. Elsewhere on the body, skin cancer is not particularly threatening, since it very rarely spreads to other organs. However, skin cancers do have a tendency to spread from the lips. Fortunately, your doctor can treat keratoses with a prescription drug called 5-fluorouracil. This drug—which is rubbed onto the surface of the skin—selectively seeks out and destroys disorganized skin cells, while sparing the normal cells. The course of treatment takes months, and at one point the affected areas ooze and look terrible. But you can apply the drug yourself, and the discomfort is a small price to pay for ridding yourself of a cancer.

Fever blisters are another type of lesion, and they can strike any age group. They're called fever blisters because fevers often seem to trigger an eruption. Actually, stress, physical trauma, and sun can trigger them just as well. The blister is caused by the herpes virus, and is called herpes type 1. A close relative of this virus is called herpes type 2, and it causes similar painful blisterlike eruptions on the genitals. There is no cure for herpes; all you can do is ease the symptoms and try to avoid incidents that might trigger the eruption. How anyone catches the virus in the first place is a topic of unresolved medical debate. However, it is generally accepted that the virus stays with you, often throughout your life, and when it isn't acting up on your lips (as in type 1) or on your genitals (as in type 2), it is thought to burrow in the nerve fibers and wait. Their dormancy in the nerve tissue is what gives rise to the speculation that stress and anxiety can trigger a herpes eruption.

If you suffer from herpes simplex, as it is officially called, you must first of all be sure to protect the lips from the sun. Next, I would recommend that you apply cool gauze compresses three times a day for fifteen minutes. You can make a good home compress solution from a quart of cool water into which you have mixed two tablespoons of salt and a cup of skim milk (or two tablespoons of powdered milk). There are medications for fever blisters on the market, but they often contain topical antihistamines that can cause allergic reactions. They also tend to retard the drying-up process, which seems counterproductive. Better to use the compresses, relax, and protect the lips from the sun. A markedly swollen lymph node under the chin commonly accompanies herpes. Don't worry, it goes away.

Finally, we come to warts, another type of lesion that can plague the lips. Warts on the lips appear as little white bumps. And let's face it, who wants to kiss a wart? Doctors can remove them fairly easily either by freezing, burning, or scraping. It's not too costly, and especially in the case of young children, I think it should be done without delay. This is not so much because the warts are dangerous as it is because other children can be shockingly cruel about such things.

Contact Dermatitis

Contact dermatitis is the term given to allergic reactions on the lips. Symptoms include redness, swelling, and, sometimes, oozing. The solution is to find out what you're allergic to and avoid it. Unfortunately, this isn't always so easy.

Common unsuspected items that often cause contact dermatitis of the lips include mangoes (whose skins contain the same chemical that's in poison ivy!), mouthwash, chewing gum, nickel in certain eating utensils (and in some tooth fillings), and the epoxy resins in some dental work.

It's extremely rare to have a reaction to lipstick or foodstuffs, since both are so thoroughly tested by manufacturers. You can sooth the dermatitis while you conduct your search for the cause by application of the compress just described in the section on lesions.

Secondary Syphilis

Most people are tipped off to syphilis infection by the presence of painless sores on the genitals. However, sometimes these initial symptoms can be overlooked, especially since they go away by themselves. Among women, where the sore may occur out of sight within the vagina, syphilis can progress through the primary stage without the victim being aware of it.

A very common symptom of secondary syphilis—the next plateau of development if the disease is untreated —is split papules. These are little white bumps that occur on both lips on each side of the mouth. It's almost as if the fissure between upper and lower lip had split each papule into an upper and lower element. Appearance of this symptom—possibly among others, including moth-eaten alopecia (hair loss) and a nonitching generalized rash over the whole body—is reason enough to call your doctor immediately. Syphilis fortunately can be treated effectively and immediately with penicillin. But don't delay.

23

Seasonal Skin Care Reminders

Spring

Spring is the season of growth, and it's also a good annual tune-up time for your skin. This is when you should remove growths, unwanted hair, and anything else that won't be covered by your bathing suit. It's also your last chance before summer for chemical peelings or dermabrasion, since you'll want to give your skin ample time to recover before heading for the beach.

Tax time is a good time to buy a sunlamp—if you don't have one already—and start your summer tan early. The sunbath section in Chapter 9, "How to Take a Bath," explains the right way to do it. Beware of majorca acne, temporary pimple flares that stem from the skin's tendency to thicken slightly with sun exposure.

This thickening, coming as it does with the first sun exposure of the year, often leads to a short bout of acne that fortunately goes away promptly. You can avoid or minimize it by preparing yourself with a sunlamp before your first day out in the sun.

Finally, irregular white blotches that appear on the skin after exposure to the sun may be caused by tinea versicolor. This is a skin fungus, harmless in almost all ways, but a nuisance because the fungus secretes a sunscreen. You can rid yourself of the fungus, and the resulting untanned white blotches, simply by bathing with Stiefel Anti-Fungal Soap.

Summer

In this season of maximum sun exposure older people in particular must be certain not to overdo it. A lifetime of too much sun leads to excessively wrinkled skin in later years. I think that everyone should use a PABA sunscreen during the summer. You'll still be able to get your tan, and twenty summers from now you'll thank yourself for your own prudence.

Summer sunshine is great medicine for acne, psoriasis, and eczema, especially in combination with saltwater. So if you suffer from these afflictions, make a point to get out in the sun as much as possible—at the beach if you can. Sunshine is so helpful for acne that you'll be able to cut down other medications and really treat the problem naturally. Again, consult the sunbath section of Chapter 9, "How to Take a Bath."

Summer is also the time for heat rash and poison ivy,

both of which can be treated with my special compress (one quart of cool water, two tablespoons of salt, and a cup of skim milk or two tablespoons of powdered milk) and applications of calamine lotion.

A final warning: Don't use deodorant soap before a sunbath. It can photosensitize your skin, and give you a painful sunburn.

Fall

This is a dangerous time for your skin, but don't panic. As the leaves fall, so does your hair, but the phenomenon is natural and no cause for alarm. The end of summertime humidity usually brings a reappearance of dry skin discomfort, so refer to Chapter 15, "Dry Skin Regimens," for relief. Without the beneficial peeling induced by the sun, acne will often start to act up again. Time to bring out the sunlamp.

Winter

Winter is a terrible time whether your skin is dry or oily. All dry skin and eczema gets worse in the winter because of the lack of humidity. Cut down on bathing and humidify your environment as best you can. Without beneficial sun exposure, acne typically gets worse or flares up seemingly from nowhere. Continue your sunlamp treatments and keep your skin clean and breathing.

Formulary

The Formulary alphabetically lists products mentioned in the text, as well as numerous others omitted because of space considerations. Product descriptions are arranged under the section headings below. Before you use a product, you are advised to consult the index, look it up in the text, and check its appropriateness for your type of skin. Please note: This is not a catalogue of every product on the market.

1. Abrasive Cleansers for Acne
2. Acne Medicines
3. Antibiotics (prescription and OTC)
4. Antifungal Medications
5. Antiparasitics
6. Astringents
7. Bath Oils
8. Bleachers
9. Creams and Lotions
10. Epiabradors
11. Masks
12. Medicated Powders
13. Psoriasis Medications

14. Shampoos (for problem hair)
15. Soaps (for acne, oily and dry skin)
16. Sun Blockers
17. Sunscreens
18. Steroids
19. Tranquilizers

1. Abrasive Cleansers for Acne

The following cleansers all work on the same principle: They contain little granules that abrade the skin
and remove dirt and oil.

Brāsivol is a grainy cleanser whose granules come in
varying sizes. You can start with fine and move up to
coarser grains.
Ionax Scrub has a pleasant lemon scent.
Komex contains granules called "scrubules" that dissolve in water.
Pernox Scrub is the granddaddy of them all. It comes in
regular and lemon-scented form.

2. Acne Medicines

Benzagel 5 and 10 are two acne gels containing benzoyl
peroxide in 5 percent and 10 percent strengths. This is a
very strong drying agent and should be used with caution. The product is marked with an expiration date.
Benoxyl 5 and 10 Lotion both contain benzoyl peroxide
in a lotion form. They are even more drying than Benzagel and should be used with caution. They also bear
an expiration date.

Betadine is a sterilizing liquid that contains iodine. It's soapy and can be used as a cleanser.

Clearasil is a good all-purpose product for mild acne.

Cort-Acne Lotion is a fairly mild preparation containing resorcin, sulphur, and alcohol.

Desquam-X 5 and 10 are similar to Benzagel but the base is slightly more sticky. Desquam-X is a strong drying agent and has an expiration date.

Fostril is a good acne gel whose active ingredient is alcohol.

Fostex Cream contains sulphur and salicylic acid. Fostex also is available in liquid form.

Klaron is a good acne lotion containing sulphur and alcohol. It has the advantage of drying clear.

Komed Lotion is particularly good for pimples and blackheads. It contains salicylic acid, sodium thiosulfate, resorcin, and alcohol.

Komed HC is the same product as Komed Lotion but has a bit of hydrocortisone added to it.

Loroxide is a flesh-tinted lotion containing benzoyl peroxide and chloroxyquinoline. It's very strong and works well.

Neutrogena Acne Gel contains witch hazel and alcohol and dries clear. It's for mild acne and is manufactured by the same people who make Neutrogena soap, noted for its purity.

PanOxyl 5 and 10 are gels containing benzoyl peroxide in lesser (5 percent) and greater (10 percent) strengths. They are very strong medicine, and are marked with an expiration date.

Persadox is a lotion that contains benzoyl peroxide.

Persa-Gel 5 and 10 contain benzoyl peroxide dispersed in acetone. They are characterized by superior absorbability and are marked with an expiration date on the package.

pHisoHex is an excellent drying cleanser particularly useful to acne sufferers. It's now a prescription item, since one of its ingredients was linked to brain damage in infants.

Postacne Lotion is for mild acne. The most active ingredient is alcohol, and it's a good product for people whose acne is clearing up.

Retin-A Brand Tretinoin is Vitamin A acid. It is a very strong product, sometimes photosensitizing, and comes in gel, cream, and towelette form.

Rezamid is a flesh-tinted acne lotion whose active ingredients are resorcin, sulphur, and alcohol. It also contains parachlorometaxylenol and is very good for mild acne.

Sulfacet-R is a very good mild acne lotion containing sodium sulfacetamide and sulfur.

Sulfacet-HC is the same product as Sulfacet-R, plus hydrocortisone.

Sulfoxyl comes in two strengths: regular and strong. Start with regular and move up to strong when you're ready.

Transact is a mild, clear acne gel containing sulfur, 40 percent alcohol, and other drying agents.

Vanoxide is an old standby in acne therapy. It dries clear, has benzoyl peroxide, and is marked with an expiration date.

Vanoxide-HC is the same product as Vanoxide with hydrocortisone added to it.

3. Antibiotics

First I'll enumerate prescription items, then over-the-counter products.

Declomycin can be highly photosensitizing.
Erythromycin is used for acne.
Nystatin is an antiyeast medication.
Penicillin doesn't help acne, but it is very good as a treatment for bacterial skin infections and syphilis.
Podophyllin is really an antiviral agent, and is used only by doctors as a treatment for warts.
Tetracycline is used for acne. It must be taken one hour before or two hours after meals lest it bind to calcium and be diverted from the skin.

Bacitracin Ointment is a good OTC, nonsensitizing superficial ointment.
Lassar's paste is a mildly antibacterial OTC paste containing zinc oxide, starch, and petrolatum.

4. Antifungal Medications

Prescription items are listed first, followed by over-the-counter medications.

Lotrimin comes in either liquid or cream form and is quite expensive.

Micatin also comes either as a cream or liquid and is also costly. Sometimes Tinactin (see below) does the job just as well.

Desenex comes in powder or cream form and is used by the army.

Salicylic Acid and Sulfur Soap is manufactured by Stiefel and is an excellent soap for removing a superficial fungus.

Tinactin comes in cream, liquid, or powder form. It's a superior product for fungus infections. Many physicians prefer the liquid form.

Whitfield's Ointment is salicylic acid and benzoic acid. It's a mild peeling ointment for fungi of the feet, and an old standby.

5. Antiparasitics

Kwell is a prescription medication that comes in cream, lotion, and shampoo form. It is usually used for scabies.

6. Astringents

Bonne Bell Ten-O-Six is an excellent astringent and an old standby.

DuBarry Astringent Lotion works well and has a nice scent.

Ionax Astringent Skin Cleaner contains alcohol, salicylic acid, and acetone. It works very well.

Ionax Lemon-Scented Foam Cleanser is very similar, with the addition of the lemon scent.

Propa-PH is a cleansing lotion whose main ingredient is alcohol.

Seba-Nil Astringent is extremely good and comes in towelettes and liquid form. The active ingredients are alcohol and acetone.

Witch Hazel is an inexpensive mild astringent lotion (also available in gel form as Neutrogena Acne Gel).

7. Bath Oils

These are for dry skin. All make your skin feel smooth and soft.

Alpha Keri has the best scent in my opinion.
Aveeno Oatmeal Bath is oilated. It's very soothing to irritated or rashy skin.
Calgon Bath Oil
Doak Oil
Johnson's Baby Oil
Kauma Bath Oil
Lubath
Neutrogena Rain Bath
Sardo
Syntex Bath Oil

8. Bleachers

These creams lighten the color of the skin.

Eldopaque is a hydroquinone titanium cream.
Eldoquin contains hydroquinone, the ingredient that lightens pigment.

9. Creams and Lotions

Aluminum chloride tincture is a prescription antiperspirant lotion sometimes recommended for sweat-related skin eruptions.

Aquacare, Aquacare/HP and *Carmol* all contain urea. This chemical is hydrophilic (it attracts and holds moisture). These products are very good for people who tend to break out but need a good lubricating lotion.

Aquaphore is analogous to hydrophilic petrolatum (see below).

Calamine lotion is mild and soothing, promotes dryness on oozing skin, and is excellent for itching and inflamed skin.

Cetaphil Lotion is soothing and cleansing and contains propylene glycol and stearyl alcohol.

Cold cream (any brand) is spermicetti white wax, mineral oil, sodium borate, and purified water. Good brand names appear below.

Cornhuskers Cream is a good hand cream used widely by men.

Doak 405 is a moisturizing cream used to plump up face wrinkles. Actually, all creams and moisturizers do the same; this one just happens to be particularly good.

Efudex is the brand name for 5-fluorouracil, a prescription cream (also a lotion) for sun-damaged skin.

Eucerine is like Nivea (see below) plus perfume.

Hydrophilic ointment is greaseless.

Hydrophilic petrolatum is greasy.

Hydrophilic petrolatum (hydrated) is a great preparation for dry skin and a good inexpensive cosmetic. It's available as Aquaphore (by Duke) and Polysorb (by Fougera).

Hydrophilic petrolatum (with water) has 30 percent water added and is a superb emollient cream for dry skin.

Jergens Hand Cream has a secret formula with a cold cream base.

Kauma Lotion is a superbly scented lotion that is hydrating in nature.

Keri comes in cream or lotion form.

Lubriderm is a lotion for dry skin and contains lanolin.

Mineral oil is an excellent makeup remover.

Neutraderm is a hypoallergenic dry skin preparation that comes in cream and lotion form.

Neutraplus cream and lotion are the same as Neutraderm with 10 percent urea added.

Neutrogena Hand Cream is a superconcentrated Norwegian formula that's particularly good for dry hands.

Nivea is a moisturizing cream made of petrolatum and water.

Petrolatum is a semisolid mixture of hydrocarbons that is very occlusive. It promotes hydration of the skin and increased moisture absorption.

Ponds Hand Cream has a cold cream base.

Purpose is a dry skin cream primarily for people who have overused acne products and need a soothing moisturizer.

Shepard's Cream Lotion is an old soothing standby that's coming back into vogue. Scented or unscented, it's a superb medication.

Shepard's Hand Cream is easy to carry as it comes in little towelettes. Contains no lanolin or mineral oil.
Unibase has a hydrophilic base.

10. *Epiabraders*

Buf-Puf is a synthetic sponge that removes the top layers of the skin.
Loofah is a natural product that does the same thing.
Tawashi also is a natural epiabrader.

11. *Masks*

Masks cleanse the face and make it feel good. In addition to the several home recipes included in the text, the following commercial preparations are good.

Max Factor Blue Mask is primarily a diagnostic tool to enable you to identify oily and dry skin areas.
Seba-Nil Cleansing Mask contains alcohol, castor oil, titanium dioxide, and granules. It is very good for acne.

12. *Medicated Powders*

Desenex is very good for people who tend to get fungus infections.
Tinactin does the same thing as Desenex.
20 Percent Fluffy Tannic Acid is a powder closely related to tea and is used to tan skin in order to reduce perspiration.

Zeasorb is primarily used to combat and dry up sweat acne on the back.

13. Psoriasis Medications

Also helpful in treating psoriasis are the dandruff shampoos (see below), Stiefel Salicylic Acid Soap, and Stiefel Polytar Soap.

Balnetar is a bath oil that contains coal tar and Alpha Keri oil.

Estar Gel is a tar gel. Tar heals rapidly dividing skin. Warning: It is a photosensitizer.

P & S Liquid contains phenol and saline. It removes scales from the scalp overnight.

Pragmatar is a very good tar preparation.

Zetar Emulsion is a tar preparation for the bath.

14. Shampoos

This section is divided into dandruff, drying, and corrective protein shampoos.

DANDRUFF SHAMPOOS

These shampoos work best if you alternate brands daily.

DHS stands for Dermatologic Hair Shampoo, a shampoo with good body-retentive quality.

DHS-T is the same as regular DHS with the addition of tar.

Excel is a pleasantly scented selenium sulfide shampoo.

Head & Shoulders contains zinc perithyon.

Iocon is a tar shampoo in a gel form.

Ionil contains salicylic acid and benzoylconium in alcohol.

Ionil-T is the same thing plus tar.

Meted is another good drying shampoo.

Pentrax is a tar shampoo.

Polytar is also a tar shampoo.

Rezamid Lotion can also be used as a shampoo.

Sebulex contains sulfur and salicylic acid.

Sebutone contains sulfur, salicylic acid, and tar.

Selsun Blue is a selenium sulfide shampoo.

Tegrin is very good and widely used.

Vanseb is a drying antidandruff shampoo.

Vanseb-T is the same product with tar added.

Zetar contains tar.

Zincon is an improved variant of Head & Shoulders.

DRYING SHAMPOOS

These shampoos are used for excessive oiliness and related acne.

Castile contains olive and rose geranium oils. Any brand is equally good.

Fostex Liquid Shampoo contains sulfur and salicylic acid and can also be used as a skin cleanser.

Ionax Shampoo

Ionil-T Shampoo contains tar, salicylic acid, and benzalkonium chloride.

Neutrogena Solid Shampoo

PanOxyl Shampoo

Pernox

CORRECTIVE PROTEIN SHAMPOOS

Protein coats the hair, making it look thicker.

Darogen
DHS Shampoo
Pantene
Protein 21
R Gen
Revlon's Milk and Honey
Vanseb

15. Soaps

The first group of products is for acne; the second is for dry skin.

SOAPS FOR ACNE OR OILY SKIN

Acne-Aid Detergent Soap contains sulfated surfactants and hydrocarbon hydrotropes.
Acnaveen Bar contains sulfur, salicylic acid, and oatmeal.
Buf-Puf Bar is mildly drying and is sold with the Buf-Puf (see Epiabraders, p. 210).
Fostex Cake contains sulfur and salicylic acid.
Fostex Liquid contains the same in liquid form.
Ivory is a mild, nonirritating soap that is good for oily skin.
Neutrogena is a very pure, mildly drying soap.
Neutrogena Acne Soap is nonalkaline and nonirritating.
pHisoHex is an excellent cleanser and disinfectant but now requires a prescription.

SAStid is a strong soap containing precipitated sulfur and salicylic acid.

Sulfur Soap contains precipitated sulfur and is milder than SAStid.

SOAPS FOR DRY SKIN

These contain a little more oil than regular soaps, making them less drying.

Alpha Keri Soap
Aveeno Bar
Basis
Caress
Dove
Kauma Soap
Lowila
Oilatum
Tone

16. Sun Blockers

These preparations completely block all sun rays.

SunStick is used on the lips and contains digalloyltrioleate.

Zinc oxide paste is white and provides complete sun protection. Unfortunately it's not cosmetically appealing.

17. Sunscreens

The current vogue in sunscreens is PABA (para-aminobenzoic acid). However, non-PABA products are often quite good.

Bain de Soleil is an old standby.

Coppertone is another old standby.

Eclipse Sunscreen Lotion contains PABA and Aquacare, so it protects and moisturizes at the same time.

Maxafil is a cream containing sinoxate and metholanthoranilate, alternatives to PABA.

Pabafilm is PABA in alcohol.

PabaGel is a very effective PABA sunscreen.

Pabanol is another good PABA sunscreen.

Presun is PABA in an alcohol-based gel.

Sea and Ski also contains PABA.

Solbar contains a screening ingredient called oxydioxydenzone.

Uval is a good sunscreen without PABA.

18. Steroids

All steroids are anti-inflammatory drugs that require a doctor's prescription. They're all closely related; these are some brand names:

Aristocort
Hytone
Kenalog
Lidex
Valisone

19. Tranquilizers

Valium comes in varying strengths and is sometimes useful in relieving itching due to stress.

Index